THE

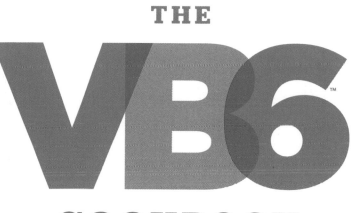

VB6

COOKBOOK

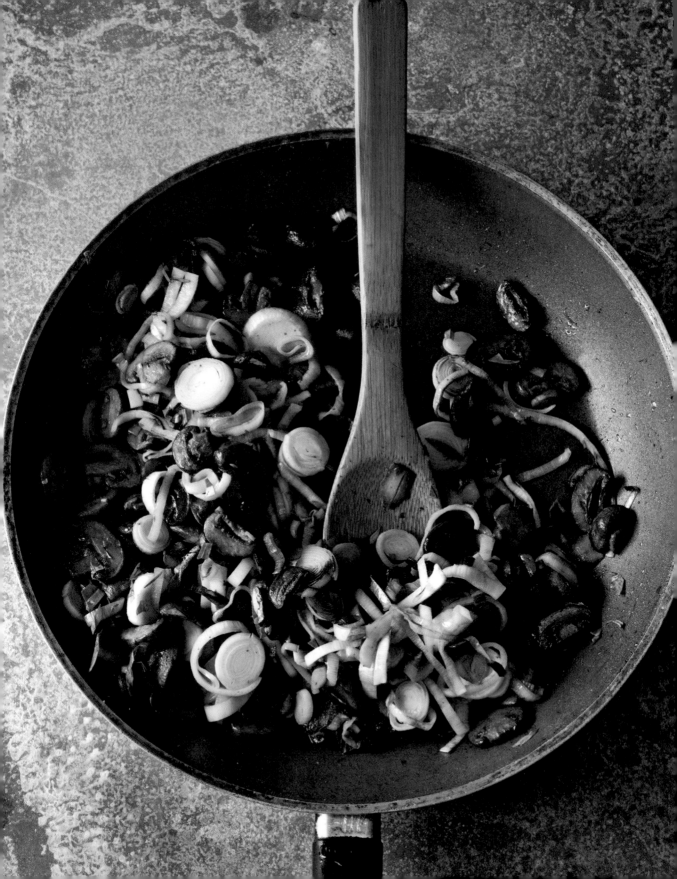

THE

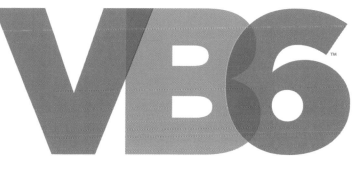

VB6™

COOKBOOK

More Than 350 Recipes for Healthy Vegan Meals All Day and
Delicious Flexitarian Dinners at Night

MARK BITTMAN

PHOTOGRAPHS BY QUENTIN BACON

CLARKSON POTTER/PUBLISHERS
NEW YORK

Published in the United States by Clarkson Potter/Publishers, an imprint of
the Crown Publishing Group, a division of Random House LLC, a Penguin
Random House Company, New York.
www.crownpublishing.com
www.clarksonpotter.com

CLARKSON POTTER is a trademark and POTTER with colophon is a
registered trademark of Random House LLC.

"VB6" and "Vegan Before Six" are trademarks of Double B Publishing, Inc.,
and may not be used without a license agreement from the owner.

Library of Congress Cataloging-in-Publication Data is available.

ISBN 978-0-385-34482-1
eBook ISBN 978-0-385-34483-8

Printed in the United States of America

Text design by La Tricia Watford
Jacket photographs by Quentin Bacon

10 9 8 7 6 5 4 3 2 1

First Edition

To everyone who makes the daily decisions,
large and small, that are changing the way we eat

—MB

CONTENTS

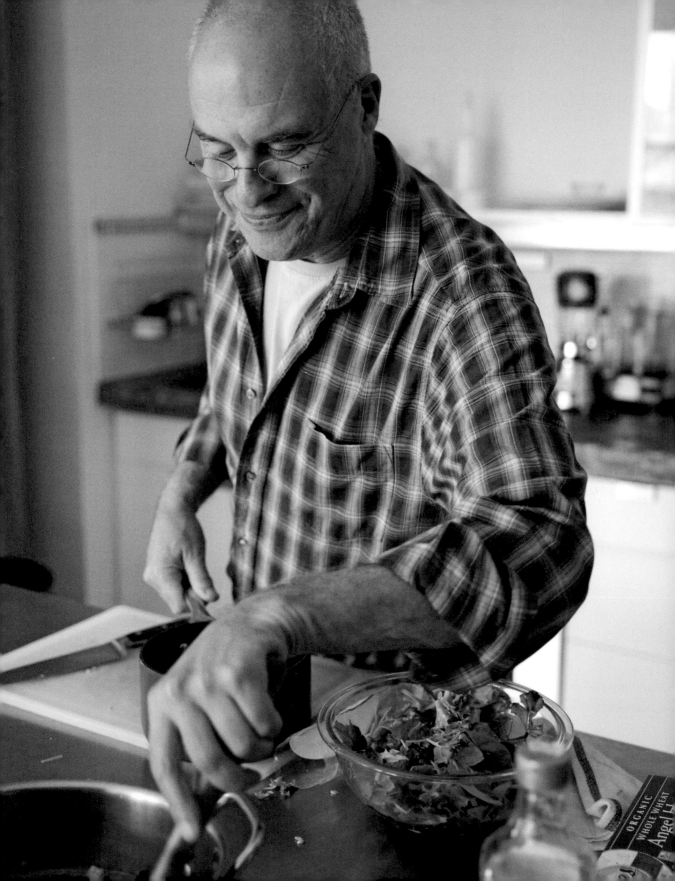

INTRODUCTION: MY STORY

I've been telling the VB6 story for seven years now, sometimes ten times in a day. I never tire of it. If anything, the passage of time makes the punch line even more powerful: Eating Vegan Before Six has turned my life around. For good.

I seem to have created a way of eating that has allowed me—a person who makes his living writing about eating and cooking—to lose weight quickly and easily, and it has now allowed me to keep it off for the better part of a decade. Over the years I've heard from many, many others that they've made similar transformations.

That's not how fad diets work.

I started VB6 on my own and on a hunch. There I was, middle aged, overweight but physically active, and sitting in my doctor's office going over the numbers. High cholesterol, check. Pre-diabetes, check. Overweight, check. Perhaps some of this will sound familiar to you too. My doctor—a man I've known and trusted for 30 years—gave me two choices: Either start taking what amounts to a lifetime of drugs to counteract the effects of obesity-related diseases, or drastically change my diet. He suggested that becoming a vegan might do the trick.

Honestly, neither sounded good. I'm against taking drugs for preventable diseases and, given the importance and variety of food in my life, veganism wasn't an option. So after planting that seed, my doctor sent me away to think of something more suitable. Instead I struck a compromise: I'd eat like an ultra-strict vegan from the time I woke up until dinnertime, and then I'd eat whatever I wanted to. And that, essentially, is VB6.

The next chapters outline exactly how you'll be eating, but ultimately there are just two rules to remember: Rule number one is that from the time you wake until 6 P.M. (or dusk, or dinnertime—any of those is fine) you eat as a strict, mindful, well-nourished vegan would: no animal products, no junk food, no highly processed food. Your daytime diet comprises only minimally processed fruits, vegetables, legumes, nuts, seeds, and whole grains. (All of this can be "negotiated," as you'll see.) Rule number two is that you do whatever you want for dinner. Including, yes, wine, beer, dessert, cheeseburgers, whatever (though, within reason) and just until dinner is over, not until midnight.

There's an obvious and important reason why the impact of VB6 is immediate and profound: It ensures that you eat more plants and less of everything else. And if there are unifying, credible points in the trustworthy research of the last 20 years, they are these: We eat too much meat; we eat too much sugar; we eat too much highly processed food (mostly grains that are metabolized as sugar); and we don't eat enough minimally processed fruits and vegetables.

After seven years of VB6 I can say with assurance that there is no downside. When I first started, it was obvious that VB6 could be in no way harmful, and therefore there was no reason not to try it. In fact the only surprises were (a) how easy it was and (b) how well it worked.

Now I look back and it seems an almost seamless transition, a move from eating an entirely undisciplined form of the Standard American Diet (yes, it is indeed SAD) to a malleable but determined pattern that took some thought during the course of the day but that paid off in both short-term pleasure—dinner every night continues to be a source of joy, and now it feels like a reward as well—and long-term health.

VB6 provides a different, more modern approach to improving the way you eat, and this book demonstrates just how flexible it can be. If your standard fare is typically American, these recipes and strategies will change that. In no time—and with little effort—you'll be consuming fewer hyper-processed foods, less industrial meat and dairy products, less sugar, and fewer chemically extracted oils; *and* you'll be consuming more natural antioxidants, micronutrients, phytochemicals, and fiber.

And all of that means you're likely to be healthier, lighter, more energetic, and in better spirits. It's difficult—no, make that impossible—to predict how a change in diet will affect any individual. That's true even for a doctor who's seen you and all your blood work. But among all the confusion and gobbledygook about health and diet that's out there, there's enough evidence to state these three things:

1 The more plants you eat, In a state as close as possible to natural, the better off you'll be.

2 The fewer highly processed foods you eat—especially highly processed grains, but other foods as well—the better off you'll be.

3 It might be presumptuous to say "the fewer animal products you eat the better off you'll be." But if you're like most Americans (and we average something like 600 pounds of animal products per person per year), you could stand to cut back, as we now know that too many animal products can be bad for your health.

VB6 will take care of all three of those things for you: increase your intake of plants and decrease your intake of highly processed foods and animal products. If you now eat a standard American diet, you will be healthier. How that "healthier-ness" will manifest itself is impossible to predict, but you may lose weight, feel better, see your blood numbers go in the right direction, sleep better, walk better, all of the above, and more. At the very least, you will probably significantly reduce your risk of chronic disease. Not bad—in fact, very good.

It's likely that you'll see those kinds of changes in two months, perhaps even sooner. But I'm not going to guarantee specific results in a set period of time because VB6 is not a conventional diet or a plan with a slew of false promises.

That's all you need to know to get started. There's no reason to continue reading if you don't want to know anything else; just dive into the recipes. This is, after all, a cookbook. (If you want to know more about why shifting the balance of your diet more toward plants and away from animals and processed foods, a great deal more detail is available in the original *VB6*.)

How long do you "stay on" VB6? For the rest of your life. It's not a "lose 21 pounds in 21 days" diet plan, but a diet in the old-fashioned sense of the word: *a way of eating*. The way you *will* eat. Period. You're not looking for a short-term quick fix, and you won't have to suffer on a restrictive and unnatural regimen for long. You are changing the way you eat for better health forever.

VB6 is a permanent commitment to a life that includes the enjoyment of good food and drink while teaching you the give-and-take necessary to either improve or maintain well-being. And when you're healthy, chances are your weight will also be okay; you may not wear the same size you did as a college freshman, but you will likely strike a weight with which you'll be comfortable. Good health, after all, is not about pounds on a scale; rather, appropriate weight is an indicator of good health. And VB6 will give you that.

EATING VB6

VB6 works in large part because a key aspect of the strategy is eating and enjoying delicious food—much of it in unlimited amounts. As someone who regularly both frequents restaurants and cooks at home I can state this without hesitation: If you cook daily, or nearly so, you'll have a far better chance of making long-lasting, positive change in your diet than if you don't.

The reasons are fundamental: Preparing your own food is the only way to know exactly what you're eating. You control the quality of the ingredients, the techniques, the seasoning, and the portion sizes. A 2010 study suggests that you can lose weight while consuming prepared foods, but that you can lose weight and eat more if you rely on minimally processed fruits and vegetables, fish, poultry, dairy, and meats.

And I don't have to tell you that gathering in the kitchen and around a familiar table are among the best ways there are to enjoy the company of friends and family, and to solidify and fortify relationships. When something is both effortless and pleasurable—as cooking will become after a while if it's not already—you're much more likely to embrace it.

Eating out is fine too, and for many people either necessary or a key part of living the good life. Familiarizing yourself with the VB6 food groups, which we'll get to soon, makes navigating a menu easy and will never leave you feeling like you're on a diet. (And remember: you aren't.)

But cooking your own food gives you so many more choices, especially for breakfast, lunch, and snacks, whereas solid, VB6 type options are harder to find out and about. The recipes here are designed to streamline preparation and help you plan ahead to make every meal as easy as grabbing takeout, if not easier. The goal is to create a lifetime of healthy habits based on a wide variety of fruits and vegetables, augmented with satisfying amounts of virtually everything else and customized to your needs and cravings. This book is designed to help you cultivate those habits, painlessly.

THE VB6 FOOD GROUPS

The best, simplest, and easiest cooking begins with good ingredients. So before getting into the recipes I'll outline how to stock your cabinets and fridge. And I've structured this discussion of the VB6 larder into three at-a-glance charts that reflect the VB6 food groups: Unlimited Foods, Flexible Foods, and Treats.

The foods in each group are selected based on how the body burns calories, provides nutrients, and stores fat. (*VB6* explains this science in great detail.) These next three chapters describe the different groups and explain how to vary your selections and use and store all the ingredients.

But by way of introduction (or review, if you're already familiar with *VB6*), Unlimited Foods are the backbone of VB6, the fruits and vegetables you can and should eat freely throughout the day. Flexible Foods include all plant-based oils and the fruits and vegetables that tend to have more protein and calories and less water by weight, the satisfying foods you eat in moderation. Treats are what you eat after 6:00 P.M., the meat, fish, poultry, eggs, and dairy ingredients you might cook every day, as well as limited amounts of the junk you'll find yourself craving less and less. These three distinctions are all you need to know to eat VB6 and switch the balance of foods in your diet away from animals and more toward plants.

HOW TO USE THIS BOOK

The VB6 Cookbook puts a collection of delicious, easy-to-make recipes into the context of a plant-based diet. The result is a prescriptive guide to changing and sustaining a lifetime of healthy and pleasurable eating. In that way, it couldn't be simpler. But a few words about the rest of the book's organization and features will make it even easier for you to grasp.

The recipes are organized to follow the course of a typical day: Breakfast, Lunch, Snacks, Dinner, and Dessert. All the ingredients are vegan until dinner, which itself is "flexitarian"—representative of a diet that's higher in plants and lower in both animal products and hyper-processed foods, but in which everything is fair game—so the recipes are based on Unlimited and Flexible Foods, with small amounts from the Treats group. Desserts are mostly vegan, with some dairy used either optionally or in very small quantities.

Many of the recipes offer tips for switching back and forth between vegan and flexitarian—that is, they can be made without or with the addition of animal products. Experimenting with these suggestions increases your repertoire exponentially and, I hope, will inspire spontaneous cooking. When you learn how to exchange ingredients to follow the seasons (or your whims!), with what looks good at the store, or simply for what you have on hand, you'll enjoy cooking and eating VB6 that much more.

To help teach by example, I offer variations after all the recipes, a hallmark of my cooking style that I believe makes cooking accessible. These are titled and appear in the index, so you can search for them by key ingredients, cuisine, and techniques. Most recipes also include a section called "More Ideas"—simple substitutions and adjustments that build on the main recipe or the variations to help you customize the recipes even more. And if you're missing a key ingredient, these tools will help you find a good substitute. Spon-taneous cooking is convenient cooking. Master this skill and you need only a handful of recipes in your repertoire to cook different dishes every day.

The majority of the recipes in this book are designed to serve four people, assuming that the dish is being prepared as a main course, along with a simple side dish or two from the "VB6 Building Blocks" chapter (page 220). If you want to serve any of these as a snack or appetizer in smaller portions, figure they'll serve eight.

WHERE'S THE NUTRITIONAL INFORMATION?

You might notice that there are no nutritional profiles in this book: no calorie counts; no "grams of" protein, or fiber, or carbs; no information about micronutrients like calcium or B vitamins. This is an intentional decision made out of the desire to let the recipes alone demonstrate the essence of what I believe is good eating for life. If you base your diet on whole, unprocessed plant foods, minimally processed fats (essential nutrients that also happen to make food taste great), and small amounts of animal foods (if you'd like), you'll be getting good nutrition. End of story. Counting calories, carbs, protein, and fat grams isn't going to get you there. Following the tenets of VB6—including portioning and proportioning foods according to the Unlimited, Flexible, and Treat groups—will. It's as simple as that.

THE UNLIMITED PANTRY

You already know that vegetables and fruit—the so-called Unlimited Foods—form the foundation of every VB6 meal and snack. But seeing them divided into groups and spread into at-a-glance tables illustrates exactly how versatile and extensive your choices are. My hope is that presenting the information this way is both convincing and reassuring; you're going to eat well, you're going to eat deliciously, and your diet is going to be as varied as ever.

VEGETABLES

Grouping vegetables by their characteristics works on many different levels. From a cooking perspective, it will help you figure out how to make substitutions easily. For example, if a recipe calls for cauliflower and you only have broccoli, chances are you can still make the dish, as you could with other, similar vegetables. Cooking times may vary, but that's pretty straightforward: less time for tender ingredients, more for firm ones. (For an all-purpose recipe, see Big-Batch Cooked Vegetables on page 227.)

You can also use these listings to expand your preferences; if you like one vegetable in the family,

chances are you'll like others. Challenge yourself to try one new vegetable every week, and eat them freely: There are only a handful that should be approached with restraint; I'll address them in "The Flexible Pantry."

I've also included a column to help you recognize seasonality—an old-fashioned concept that's made a big comeback. Of course produce is grown and shipped around the globe, so you can always find what you want, especially vegetables. But use this part of these guides for when you're buying close to home or regionally.

And remember that fresh produce isn't your only option. I always keep a few bags of frozen vegetables on hand; spinach and other greens, winter squashes, peas, green beans, carrots, edamame, and corn are all good. (Even many others are not at all bad in a pinch.) Canned vegetables and fruits are another matter; stick to tomatoes (see the sidebar at left), roasted peppers, and beans, which are on the Flexible Foods list. To avoid bisphenol A—BPA, a potentially toxic chemical found in some plastic containers and the linings of some cans—try to find these foods in jars or cans that are labeled "BPA Free."

CANNED TOMATOES

I'm a fan of the canned tomato, which is convenient, inexpensive, and better than out-of-season fresh ones. Look for whole plum (Roma, usually) or San Marzano varieties. Canned diced tomatoes are a little less hassle, though their quality can vary greatly. Since I like bits of tomatoes in my sauces and stews, I rarely use crushed or pureed tomatoes, but try in these recipes if you prefer. And I always avoid anything with additives, sugars, or seasonings.

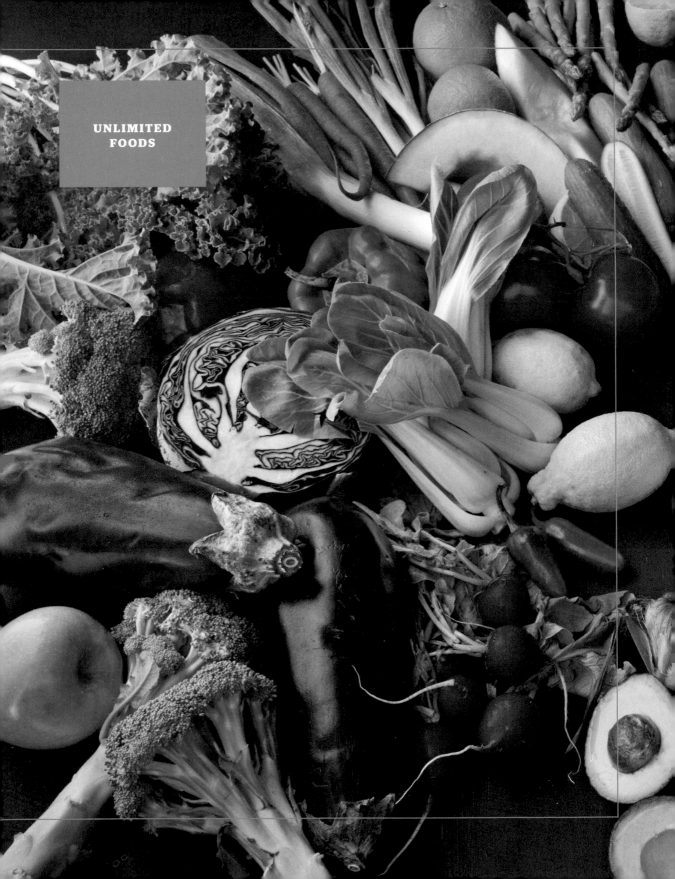

UNLIMITED
FOODS

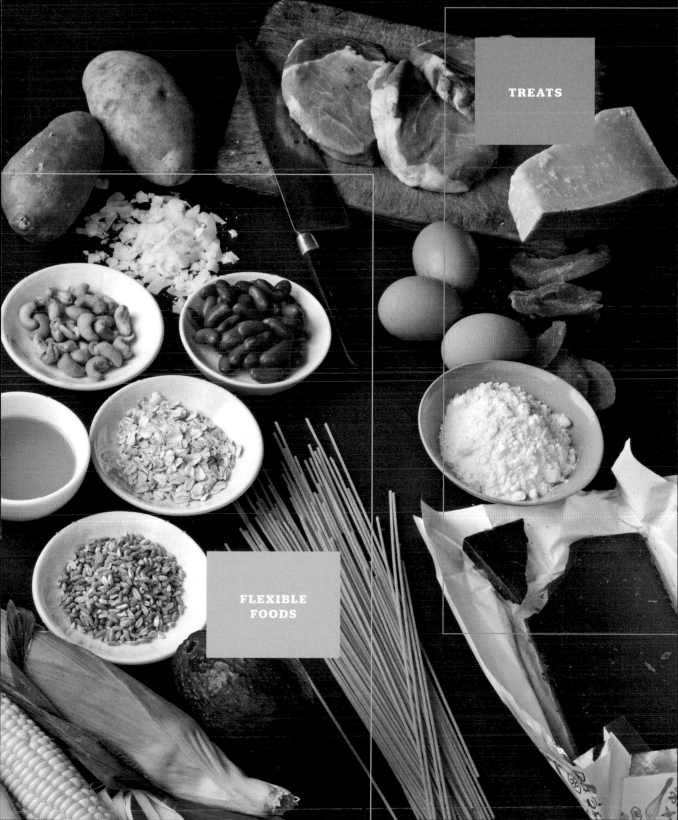

TREATS

FLEXIBLE
FOODS

UNLIMITED VEGETABLES

VEGETABLE GROUP	WHAT THEY ARE	BEST TIME OF YEAR	HOW TO STORE	BEST WAYS TO PREPARE
LEAFY (all sorts of greens and cabbage-like vegetables)	From tender to sturdy: all lettuces and salad greens, watercress, spinach, dandelion, chicory, endive chard, escarole, bok choy (and other Asian greens), kale, collards, broccoli raab, broccoli, cauliflower, Brussels sprouts, cabbages.	All year round, but locally raised lettuces are generally best in spring and fall.	Keep salad greens in a spinner (see page 224); others should be refrigerated, wrapped loosely in plastic or stored directly in one of the bins. Many sturdy kinds will keep a week; cabbages can last a few weeks.	Eat raw; or microwave, steam, boil, sauté or stir-fry, braise, or roast. (You can even grill or broil them.)
NIGHTSHADES (the fruits of the vegetable world)	Perhaps my favorite group: eggplant, bell peppers, chiles, tomatoes, tomatillos.	Summer. They're available almost all the time but quality can vary wildly. (Use dried chiles and tomatoes in winter if you can't find fresh.)	Keep tomatoes and tomatillos on the counter until they're ripe, then eat or cook them right away. The others will keep for at least a week in the refrigerator.	Eggplant isn't good raw but all the others are. Otherwise, microwave, steam, sauté or stir-fry, braise, roast, or grill or broil.
STALK OR STEM VEGETABLES	The catchall group at first glance, but there are similarities: celery, fennel, asparagus, mushrooms, artichokes, cardoons, kohlrabi, cactus.	All year round for mushrooms and celery; for the others, spring into summer.	Refrigerate these, wrapped loosely in plastic or stored directly in one of the bins. You can put mushrooms in a paper bag so they won't get slimy; use precious specialty mushrooms almost immediately to protect your investment.	Eat raw (yes, even artichokes); thinly sliced is best; otherwise, microwave, steam, sauté or stir-fry, braise, roast, or grill or broil.
EDIBLE-POD LEGUMES	More varieties available all the time: green and wax beans, snow peas, snap peas.	Spring for the peas; summer for the beans.	Refrigerate, wrapped loosely in plastic or stored directly in one of the bins. Eat within a few days, even if they don't look so bad because their flavor dissipates quickly, especially tender snow peas.	You can eat these raw if you chop or slice them thin, but they're generally better after brief cooking: microwave, steam, boil, sauté or stir-fry, or braise; green and wax beans are also good roasted.

VEGETABLE GROUP	WHAT THEY ARE	BEST TIME OF YEAR	HOW TO STORE	BEST WAYS TO PREPARE
ROOT VEGETABLES AND TUBERS	All are entirely interchangeable: radishes, jícama carrots, beets, celery root, turnips, rutabaga, parsnips.	These are workhorses throughout the year, since they keep for a long time. Most are harvested in fall and winter except for radishes, which are best in spring and fall but available always.	The key with these is to keep them chilled. Loose in a bin in the refrigerator is fine. Radishes dry out faster than others. Once trimmed and peeled you can keep sliced root vegetables and tubers in a bowl of water in the fridge for several days.	Raw, especially when thinly sliced. Radishes are surprisingly good cooked, but note that they get tender in a flash. For the others you can microwave, steam, boil, sauté or stir-fry, braise, or roast. To grill, cook over indirect or low heat with the lid on.
SUMMER SQUASHES	The tender, quick-cooking, more watery squashes: zucchini, yellow squash, pattypan, and other specialty varieties.	They're the classic summer vegetable.	Refrigerate zucchini wrapped loosely in plastic or in one of the bins. They start losing flavor after several days but usually keep for at least a week.	They're good raw, especially sliced thinly. Otherwise, you can microwave, steam, sauté or stir-fry, braise, roast, grill, or broil.
WINTER SQUASHES	A big family of firm, long-storing vegetables that includes pumpkin, butternut, acorn, spaghetti, kabocha, delicata.	Harvested in fall and kept through winter.	Store winter squashes in a cool, dry place other than the fridge. (I sometimes just leave them out on the table or counter as a decoration.) They should keep for months.	You can eat them raw, but marinate them in dressing first. Or you can microwave, steam, sauté or stir-fry, braise, or roast.
AROMATICS	Aromatics are the staples that make everything else taste better (and are sometimes good on their own): onions, garlic, ginger, shallots, and leeks. Use them alone or in combination.	These are available all year long.	Store onions, ginger, shallots, and garlic at room temperature if you're going to use them within a week or so; otherwise put them in the fridge. Leeks should always be in the fridge, either loosely wrapped in plastic or in a bin.	They're good raw but strong-tasting. The best way to develop their flavor is by sautéing or stir-frying. But you can also braise, roast, grill, or broil onions and leeks.

(continues)

VEGETABLE GROUP	WHAT THEY ARE	BEST TIME OF YEAR	HOW TO STORE	BEST WAYS TO PREPARE
SPROUTS	Seeds with shoots, commonly made from alfalfa, lentil, wheat, radish, or soy and mung beans. Microgreens, which are teeny lettuce spouts, are also increasingly popular—and dear.	Commercially, most are available year round, since they literally can be grown in a closet. Microgreens used to be spring only, but now they're grown in greenhouses so you see them all sorts of times of the year.	Wrap them loosely in plastic or a towel and keep in the fridge. But eat them right away because they lose their crunch fast.	Raw is really best for most of these, except for the sturdier bean sprouts, which are also good quickly steamed or stir-fried, or tossed into a pot of soup at the last minute.

FRUIT

Fruit is my go-to food when I'm packing for a trip or dashing out the door for a long day. And I always try to incorporate at least one piece into my dessert. (Often, in fact, a bowl of cut-up fruit *is* my dessert.) And remember, fruit is not just for snacking: It's fantastic in salads, on the grill, or roasted with nuts and spices. In many parts of the world, fruit—in particular melons and tropicals like mango and papaya—is frequently eaten sprinkled with salt, ground red chile, and a squeeze of lime.

So have at 'em. Using fruit as a cooking ingredient will only expand the variety of color, flavors, textures, and nutrients in your meals. In the list that follows I've again grouped the produce according to similarities and provided some ideas for how to use them.

Almost all fruit qualifies as an unlimited food for VB6ers. You can eat freely from the list that follows, especially if it keeps you from reaching for junk food or candy. Don't let anyone tell you that fruit is too carbohydrate or sugar heavy; there are lots of reasons why you should eat it whenever you want it. Fruit is high in fiber, vitamins, and micro-nutrients. Choosing it over salty or sweet snacks is always the better choice.

Like vegetables, fresh fruit is always best in season and bought locally. But since the local season is usually short, you're going to wind up buying some frozen and some from far away. On these pages I've outlined how their seasonality ebbs and flows. Fruit is even easier to substitute for than vegetables, which works to your advantage and helps give you plenty of options all year long.

UNLIMITED FRUITS

FRUIT GROUP	WHAT THEY ARE	BEST TIME OF YEAR	HOW TO STORE	BEST WAYS TO PREPARE
CITRUS	Oranges, grapefruit, lemons, limes, tangerines, mandarins, clementines, tangelos.	Winter is the best time for these fruits, and that's when you need to fill in the most gaps, so citrus can be a lifesaver.	If you're going to eat these in a day or two, leave them out. Any longer than that, better stick them in the fridge. They'll keep for weeks.	Peel and toss the segments into salads or chop them to make fresh salsas. You can also stew, stir-fry, or roast them. Or cut the fruit in half after peeling and grill or broil them.
MELONS	Watermelon, cantaloupe, honeydew, casaba, and lots of heirloom and specialty varieties.	Summer is best for these.	The thicker the skin, the better they'll keep. Check them frequently and eat them when they smell fruity but are still firm. Or refrigerate them at that point to prolong their life a few days.	Raw, but you can also roast, grill, or broil thick slices. They're amazing cooked fast, over high heat:
STONE AND TREE FRUITS	Apples, pears, peaches, nectarines, apricots, plums, cherries, figs.	Summer for most; fall for apples and pears. Plums straddle the seasons in most places.	Most are quite fragile and last only a couple days after ripening. Let them soften at room temperature, then put them in the fridge.	All are great raw; but this group takes particularly well to cooking. Try poaching, stewing, sautéing or stir-frying, roasting or baking, slow oven-drying, grilling, or broiling.
TROPICALS	Bananas and plantains, mango, pineapple, papaya, kiwi, and other exotic fruits.	Bananas are ubiquitous year-round, and pineapples nearly so. The others come in and out of season in various locations.	Leave tropical fruits at room temperature until they ripen and get soft, then move them to the fridge to prolong their life a few days.	Terrific raw and mixed with other fruit in salads. But you can also poach, stew, sauté or stir-fry, roast, oven-dry, grill, or broil.
BERRIES	Strawberries, blue-berries, blackberries, raspberries. (I count grapes in this group, too, since you eat them like berries.)	Spring and summer are best; otherwise buy frozen berries. Grapes are best in summer and fall (and don't come frozen).	Since these are so fragile and precious, better eat them as soon as you can. Keep them in the fridge until then.	Cooking makes them jammy fast. You can stew, microwave, sauté or stir-fry, roast, or oven-dry.

CONDIMENTS AND SEASONINGS

Sometimes vegetables need nothing more than salt and pepper, and fruit rarely even needs that. But you can have some fun by sprucing up a simply cooked dish or turning the flavors into something completely new simply by adding herbs, spices, vinegars, or condiments.

With the exception of fresh herbs, these are true pantry items. They keep very well, so stock as many as you think you'll use and enjoy. Buy the best quality you can afford and consider it an investment. (Your meals will still be less expensive than eating out.) If you have several of these on hand you'll be more inclined to cook; for example, they can make a plate of simply grilled fish and vegetables taste different every time. And that will help you eat better and sustain the principles of VB6 for the long haul.

UNLIMITED CONDIMENTS AND SEASONINGS

CONDIMENT GROUP	WHAT THEY ARE	HOW TO STORE	BEST WAYS TO USE
SALT AND PEPPER	The necessities. For salt, kosher is best; it's not iodized like table salt and is coarser. I skip the trendy, expensive stuff but like to have sea salt for last-minute sprinkling. For pepper, invest in a grinder, then buy whole black peppercorns and grind as you go.	Handy by the stove and on the table. Keep backup supplies in the pantry.	The connection between salt and high blood pressure is individual so check with your doctor if this is an issue. The recipes in this book call for small amounts in the ingredient lists and encourage you to taste and adjust the seasoning before serving.
FRESH HERBS	I divide them into two categories: mild, which you can use more liberally; and intense, which are best used judiciously. In the mild category are cilantro, basil, parsley, mint, dill, chervil, and chives. The strong ones include oregano, sage, marjoram, rosemary, tarragon, thyme, and lavender. In general use up to 1 cup of chopped leaves from mild herbs, and start with no more than 1 tablespoon of leaves from strong herbs.	Keep herbs in the fridge one of two ways: in a vessel of water, like cut flowers; or wrapped in a damp towel and put in a plastic bag or one of the bins. They'll keep for a few days, but are best used sooner rather than later.	Try to have at least one fresh herb handy at all times. Parsley is the most durable and versatile, and it's available year round. For the most flavor, add herbs toward the end of cooking or as a garnish. Or make pesto (herb puree) and herb sauces, and use to boost flavor.

CONDIMENT GROUP	WHAT THEY ARE	HOW TO STORE	BEST WAYS TO USE
DRIED HERBS	The only ones that taste good are dill, oregano, marjoram, sage, thyme, and rosemary; the rest have little—or worse, musty—flavor.	Don't leave them out in the light; keep them in a cupboard so their flavor stays strong.	Use dried herbs toward the beginning of the dish when you're about to add liquid so they don't burn. They work well in stews, sauces and marinades, and dressings for times you don't have fresh. Start with a teaspoon and go from there.
SPICES AND SPICE BLENDS	There's literally a world of them. Some of my favorites are smoked paprika, cumin, cinnamon, coriander, curry powder, chili powder, garam masala, and mustard seeds. See pages 244–245 for some more ideas.	Treat like dried herbs: in a cool, dark place in a sealed container. Spices keep so well, for so long, you'll need to stock up only once or twice a year.	Aficionados can buy whole spices and toast and grind them before each use. But pre-ground are fine and what I call for in the recipes. It's best to warm spices along with the aromatics or add them during cooking; their flavor improves with a little heat as long as you don't burn them.
DRIED CHILES	There are literally hundreds, which range from mild (like poblanos and New Mexican green chiles) to hot (like Thai, cayenne, and serrano) to fiery (like habanero). Some—like chipotle and ancho—are smoked before drying and taste like it. You've got to try and taste to see what you prefer.	Treat like dried herbs and spices: Store them in a cool, dark place in a sealed container.	You can buy dried chiles pre-ground or whole, which like spices should be toasted before grinding. You can also add whole chiles to a dish as it cooks and then fish them out later. Good for spiking soups, stews, sauces, and stir-fries with heat and/or smokiness. Taste and add as you go; the intensity varies with the type of chile.
VINEGARS	Try as many as you like and can afford. My favorites are sherry vinegar (one of the strongest), rice vinegar (the mildest and best for Asian-flavored dishes), and balsamic vinegars (both white and the traditional aged dark kind). Red or white wine vinegar is handy, too. Always buy the best quality you can find and afford.	They're fine in the pantry and can be used even if they get a little cloudy on the bottom.	A splash of vinegar will brighten any dish. Use them in salad dressings, stews, and marinades. They're strong enough that usually no more than 1 or 2 tablespoons is all you need, and sometimes I even cut them with a little water to reduce their intensity. The obvious use is for dressing salads, but they're also good in soups or stews and for last-minute garnishing as you would use a squeeze of citrus.

(continues)

CONDIMENT GROUP	WHAT THEY ARE	HOW TO STORE	BEST WAYS TO USE
MUSTARD	Dijon-style or whole-grain mustard (or both) is a must. Avoid those with a lot of added sugar, like honey mustard. Taste a few and see what you like; some are more acidic than others.	Refrigerate after opening.	Use in marinades, salad dressings, and sauces. Mustard can add a slight spice that completely changes a dish with just 1 tablespoon.
SALSAS	To make your own see page 236 and page 239. Or get the good stuff in jars, not cans. And make sure it doesn't have added fat or chemicals.	Refrigerate after opening.	Eat salsa on its own as a side dish or use it as a marinade, salad dressing, or base for a sauce. I also top tofu scrambles (see pages 71–72) with a spoonful of salsa.
BOTTLED SAUCES	Hot sauces, ketchup, barbecue sauce, srirachas, sambals, classic Southern-style and Caribbean bottled pepper sauces, and the like. Industrially made pouring sauces tend to be loaded with high fructose corn syrup so try to either make your own or seek out the kind that are minimally processed and sweetened with table sugar—and then use them judiciously.	Refrigerate after opening, unless you're going to use them fast.	I tend to use these as ingredients in sauces or other dishes rather than adding them at the table, but you can certainly do that, too.
SOY SAUCE	Made from fermented toasted wheat and soy beans. Nothing adds savory flavor faster. Just read the label to be sure you get the real deal and not flavored water. There shouldn't be more than a handful of ingredients.	This keeps fine in the pantry for months, though it may thicken slightly and intensify as the water evaporates from it.	You expect to use soy sauce in stir-fries but it's also a delicious addition to marinades, soups, and stews to round out and balance other flavors, as salt does. You can also use it as a table seasoning with Asian-style dishes.

THE FLEXIBLE PANTRY

I grouped foods as "Flexible"—rather than unlimited—not because they're "bad" for you (in fact, many are extremely beneficial) but because they have high calorie density: Per ounce (or gram) of weight they have more calories and less water. This is where the handful of starchy or fatty fruits and vegetables live, along with beans, whole grains, rice, whole-grain pastas, oils, nuts and seeds, and minimally processed sources of vegetable protein like non-dairy milks and tofu. (Have a look at the section that follows about fats [see page 31], the most calorie-dense flexible foods.)

If weight loss is a primary concern for you, the way you eat Flexible Foods is really important because it'll probably determine whether you lose weight or maintain it. In other words, if you get to a point in your new eating habits when you're not losing as much weight as you'd like to—and assuming you're being quite disciplined in your VB6 practice—try cutting back on your portions of Flexible Foods. If you're at your desired weight, you can indulge in more Flexible Foods and probably maintain it more or less permanently.

To reduce the amount of Flexible Foods you eat, consider either beans *or* rice for lunch most days, not both; think of a green salad or a chopped salad (unlimited) topped with one or the other. When you need an afternoon snack, reach for an apple or some carrots instead of nuts.

Remember that Flexible Foods are necessary and important; they're loaded with vitamins, antioxidants, fiber, and other nutrients essential for good health. So you can enjoy them all, but remember that the bulk of what you put on your plate at any given meal—and what you primarily snack on throughout the day—should come from the Unlimited Foods group.

FLEXIBLE FRUITS AND VEGETABLES

What makes this short list of produce calorie dense is either their starch or their fat content. (Unlimited fruits and vegetables tend to be made up of mostly water, fiber, and fructose.) These fruits and vegetables are just as nutritious (if not more nutritious) as any other, but their calorie density makes it important to consume them more conservatively.

> ### BUY ORGANIC—OR NOT?
> I'm asked this all the time and my answer is simple: Buy more fruits and vegetables. Period. If you have access to locally raised produce, all the better. If you can find and afford the stuff that's organically raised and certified, then go for it. Your choice will help minimize the use of pesticides—and the rate at which you ingest them, second-hand poisons. But don't let perfection be the enemy of good and skip vegetables and fruits just because organic varieties aren't available.

FLEXIBLE FRUITS AND VEGETABLES

VEGETABLE GROUP	WHAT THEY ARE	BEST TIME OF YEAR	HOW TO STORE	BEST WAYS TO PREPARE
AVOCADOS	They range from tiny to melon size, with all types of smooth or nubby skins, but only a fraction make it to our markets—mostly Hass and Fuerte varieties.	April through September for those from California; the ones from Florida start and end a little later.	Buy avocados rock hard and they'll ripen on the counter in a few days, then move them to the fridge where they'll keep for up to a week. Once they are cut, add a little citrus juice or vinegar to postpone the inevitable browning.	Almost always best raw. Adding them to salads is a good way to stretch their flavor; or mash or puree. If you want to cook them, try grilling.
CORN	The grain that eats like a vegetable. The kernels may be yellow, white, or a mixture. You can also find heirloom varieties of all different colors at farmers' markets.	Summer. But frozen corn is a good substitute in most recipes.	Refrigerate fresh corn in its husk. It's usually fine for a week but starts getting starchier after a day or two. Frozen corn will keep well for months.	Raw fresh corn is great in salads. Grill whole cobs, then husk them; or husk them first and boil, steam, or roast. For kernels, microwave, sauté or stir-fry, puree, braise, or roast.
PEAS	Shell peas, snow peas, sugar snap peas.	In-shell peas are a treat (and a pain to extract), but they're only available for a small window in spring; otherwise frozen are fine. For the others, spring is best, though you sometimes see them in late winter and into summer.	Put fresh peas loosely in plastic and store in the refrigerator. Use them ASAP. Frozen peas will keep well for months.	If they're really fresh, eat them raw. Otherwise, microwave, steam, sauté or stir-fry, or quickly braise.
ALL POTATOES	There are three categories: Starchy (like Russet), waxy (like red or fingerling), all-purpose (which are in-between, like Yukon Gold). Sweet potatoes and yams are not closely related (and are more nutritious).	Potatoes are available all year long because they store well. But if you ever have a chance, try them just-out-of-the-ground; they're amazing.	Store in a dark, cool, dry spot (the fridge is fine, in a bottom drawer) for weeks or even months.	The easiest is to toast whole in their skins, without any foil. Or cut or slice and grill, roast, boil, steam, or braise. You even can grate and stir-fry them and they're always good deep fried—as a treat of, course.

VEGETABLE GROUP	WHAT THEY ARE	BEST TIME OF YEAR	HOW TO STORE	BEST WAYS TO PREPARE
COCONUT	Fresh is a hassle but delicious. Otherwise, buy unsweetened dried, either grated, shredded, or in larger ribbons.	Year-round for both. Fresh is usually only available in specialty markets.	Fresh coconuts keep for weeks or even months in a cool dry spot. Store dried in the pantry if you go through it quickly, otherwise in the freezer. You'll smell when it loses freshness, usually in less than 6 months.	Good raw or toasted over low heat in a dry skillet or the oven.
TROPICAL TUBERS	The starchy and sometimes fibrous underground vegetables of warm climates; yuca (cassava), malanga, and taro are most common. Try some if you haven't before.	Different kinds come in and out of season throughout the year. Some are available frozen, which is a convenient way to go.	Refrigerate or keep a cool, dry, dark spot. Some do not keep as well as potatoes, so use them relatively quickly.	Just like potatoes: boil, bake in their skins, roast, fry, or braise in sauce.
100 PERCENT FRUIT AND VEGETABLE JUICES	I'm talking only about juice that you (or someone else) makes by running whole food through a juicer or blender. No processing. No additives. No sweeteners. Flexible juice can be made from any fruits or vegetables, alone or in combination. Commercially made bottled and frozen juices count as treats and are not much better for you than soda.	Whenever the fruits and vegetables made from them are at their best.	Store in the refrigerator for up to a few days.	Judicious sipping or mixing with water and teas, marinades, dips, soups, sauces, and for saucing up stir-fries.

BEANS

I eat beans almost daily and you probably will, too. The protein and fiber will help keep you full for a long time; they're easy to cook, store, and use; and boredom is never an issue, since there are literally hundreds of kinds and forms. There are nuances of flavor and texture from bean to bean, but they all respond the same way to basic techniques so I've grouped them by the range of time it takes to cook them.

Dried beans are good a year or more in your pantry. They tend to lose moisture as they sit, which means older beans take longer to cook; that's why I've put broad ranges in the chart that follows. Frozen beans keep for a few months; fresh must be cooked within a week or so. For everything you need to know about how to cook and eat them from scratch, from frozen, or from cans, see the master recipe on page 232.

FLEXIBLE BEANS

BEAN GROUPS	COMMON TYPES	COOKING TIMES	BEST WAYS TO USE
QUICKEST COOKING	Frozen beans: lima, edamame (in or out of their shells), fava, and black-eyed peas	5 to 20 minutes	This group cooks up firm, intact, and chewy, so they're great for salads, stir-fries, or soups when you want distinctive texture.
QUICK COOKING	Lentils (all kinds); split peas; split pigeon peas; adzuki and mung beans; other beans and split peas used for dals; and fresh beans like black-eyed peas or chickpeas	20 to 40 minutes	Lentils and adzuki are available in cans; otherwise you've got to cook them from dried. These go from firm and intact to soft and creamy fast, so they're perfect for dals, soups, stews, and purees or dips. But if you stop cooking them before they disintegrate, these beans are also great for cold or warm salads.
MEDIUM COOKING	Black, black-eyed peas, cannellini, cranberry, flageolet, Great Northern, kidney, lima, navy, pink, pinto, soy (black or white), and many others	40 to 90 minutes	Most canned beans come from this group. If you cook them yourself, you choose whether you want them firm and intact or soft and creamy. See the row above for how to use them.
LONG COOKING	Chickpeas, fava beans (the whole, mature, dried kind), gigantes, and large lima and butter beans	1 to 2 hours, and sometimes longer	Also available canned. Not surprisingly these are the heartiest of the bunch—perfect for stews, chilis, soups, or purees and dips.

BROWN RICE AND WHOLE GRAINS

If you don't have much experience with whole grains, you're in for a pleasant surprise; if you're familiar, then I hope this section inspires you to explore even more. They bear little resemblance to their "white" counterparts—Treats, in the world of VB6—which lose fiber and nutrients in the milling process. This also means brown rices and whole grains retain their nutty flavor and the wonderful texture that you'll love.

These valuable foods have almost as many cooking options as do beans, so again I've grouped them by cooking time to encourage you to try different kinds. Store brown rice and whole grains in tightly sealed containers in the pantry or, if you're slow to use them, keep in the fridge or freezer to prolong their freshness. For all you need to know about how to cook and serve grains, see the recipe on page 230.

FLEXIBLE WHOLE GRAINS

GRAIN GROUP	COMMON TYPES	COOKING TIMES	BEST WAYS TO USE
SUPER-QUICK COOKING	Whole wheat couscous (technically a pasta that cooks like a grain), bulgur (pre-cooked cracked wheat), rolled oats, amaranth	10 to 20 minutes	Porridges, pilafs, salads, grain burgers and griddle cakes, and even desserts. Add to soups, stews, stir-fries, or pastas. Or just eat them plain as a side dish.
QUICK COOKING	Short-grain brown rice, quinoa, steel-cut oats, cracked wheat, millet, farro, freaka, cornmeal and grits (see *hominy,* below), kasha (toasted buckwheat groats), and buckwheat groats. (Pearled barley would be in this category but is technically a "white" food.)	20 to 30 minutes	These have more heft than those above but can be used in the same ways.
MEDIUM COOKING	Long-grain brown rices, hulled (whole-grain) barley, oat groats, wild rice	30 to 60 minutes	These are particularly good when you want to keep the grains intact, with tender interiors that retain the slightest chew.
LONG COOKING	Wheat and rye berries, spelt, kamut	1 to 2 hours	Seriously chewy; perfect for hearty grain salads, pilafs, soups, and stews and even stir-fries.
LONGEST COOKING	Hominy (also known as posole) made from both white and blue corn. It must be hulled and processed to eat, so technically this form of corn isn't a whole grain, but it still has a fair amount of fiber.	Anywhere from 2 to 4 hours (a little less if soaked first)	This is the one grain you can also buy canned, which is very convenient; just drain and rinse well before using in stews, soup, stir-fries. (The classic Mexican soup known as posole is based on hominy.)

WHOLE-GRAIN PASTAS AND NOODLES

Although more processed than whole grains, these are considered Flexible Foods because they have more fiber and nutrients—including protein—than white pastas and noodles. (See page 40 in the Treat Pantry.) You'll like the slightly grainy texture and deep flavor of these noodles.

To help you use pastas and noodles interchangeably in recipes I've again slotted them into groups. The recipes in the book all give specific cooking instructions, but what follows is some general information for improvising your own pasta and noodle dishes.

FLEXIBLE PASTAS AND NOODLES

GROUP	COMMON TYPES	COOKING TIMES	BEST WAYS TO USE
ITALIAN PASTA	Made from whole ground durum wheat into traditional cut and long shapes like shells, rigatoni, farfalle, spaghetti, linguini, fettuccini, or lasagna noodles.	Varies depending on the thickness and type, but the range is 5 to 12 minutes in a pot of salted boiling water.	After cooking toss with sauce, or stir-fry with other ingredients; use in soups and stews. Pasta salads are best at room temperature; the noodles aren't as tough as they are cold.
ASIAN NOODLES	Worth seeking out whole-grain types, like soba (from buckwheat); whole wheat udon or lo mein; brown rice noodles of varying thicknesses. If you can't find what you want, use long wheat pastas.	The finer ones only require soaking in boiling or hot water for anywhere from 5 to 20 minutes. Others cook like other pasta but generally take as little as 3 minutes to become tender.	Once they're cooked, you can hold them in cold water for up to 1 hour to keep them from sticking together. Good for soups, stews, salads, and stir-fries.
SPECIALTY PASTAS	Made from ground chickpeas, corn, quinoa, farro, or kamut. Many are gluten free.	Cook in salted boiling water but start checking after 3 minutes because generally they become tender quickly.	Take into account their particular flavors and textures. Some will be sweeter, others nuttier; most tend to be stickier than traditional noodles.

A WORD ABOUT BAKING INGREDIENTS

There are only a few absolute necessities when it comes to VB6 baking: whole wheat flour (either all-purpose or pastry), baking soda, baking powder, and yeast. White flour is listed in the Treat Pantry (see page 40). If you're a regular baker and want to explore other worlds of VB6-style whole-grain sweet and savory baking, or if you have gluten intolerance, I encourage you to try brown-rice flour, masa harina, chickpea flour, and nut flours.

OILS

Ounce for ounce, these are the most calorie-dense Flexible Foods but also the most flavorful. And despite what you may have heard, you need fats to live. Fats also help satisfy you and keep you feeling full. So if you think eliminating fat from your diet is a good idea, forget it.

That said, if you want to control how fast or slow you lose weight—or if you're trying to maintain—changing your fat intake can have an impact. The recipes in this book call for what I consider is a moderate amount of healthy oils and balance both flavor and quantity. Adjust the amount at will, keeping in mind that you need at least some fat in your diet and that even a little can greatly enhance the eating experience.

Store oils you use often at room temperature in an airtight bottle or jar in small quantities, ideally in a dark, cool place. Keep oils you don't use much (or any large quantities you might have) in the fridge. When oils start to go rancid they have a distinctly "off" smell and taste that indicate it's time to replace them.

FLEXIBLE OILS

GROUP	BEST TYPES	BEST WAYS TO USE
OLIVE OIL	When I say this I always mean "extra-virgin olive oil," which is cold pressed and minimally processed. You'll use this oil for almost everything, and with its high concentration of monosaturated fats it's considered among the healthiest. The country of origin is less important; even relatively inexpensive olive oils can be quite flavorful. Avoid oils that are light, either in color or in name.	Everything means everything: dressings, cold sauces, marinades, sautéing and stir-frying, roasting, grilling, and broiling. You can use it before, during, and after cooking. With really good-tasting oils, last-minute drizzling is terrific, since you don't lose any flavor to the heating process.
"VEGETABLE" OIL	This is what to use when you want milder flavor. Vegetable oil is in quotations here because when I call for vegetable oil in this book, I mean true oils squeezed from vegetables (or fruits or seeds, to be exact) rather than the highly refined stuff labeled simply "vegetable oil" (which is highly processed from soybeans and/or corn). The best vegetable oils are grapeseed, sunflower, safflower, and peanut. These are high-heat, polyunsaturated oils with subtle differences in taste so they're relatively interchangeable. I don't use canola oil—it tastes bitter and sticky to me—but I know a lot of people do, so go ahead and use it if you can find one that is minimally processed.	Versatile and useful especially for cooking dishes from Asian cuisines when you don't want the distinct flavor of olive oil. Use for dressings, sauces, sautéing and stir-frying, roasting, grilling, or broiling, and those occasional times when you pan- or deep-fry.
OTHER OILS	These are the intensely flavored oils squeezed from intensely flavored nuts and seeds. Sesame oil (made from toasted seeds and dark in color) is the oil I use most from this group, but I like hazelnut and walnut oils too. Others you might want to try: almond, avocado, or hemp.	Generally these oils are sensitive to heat and best used for cold dishes, dips and cold sauces, and drizzling.

NUTS AND SEEDS

Nuts and seeds are a valuable component of VB6 eating, for they are excellent sources of protein, unsaturated fat, vitamins, fiber, and other nutrients. Like the other Flexible Foods, they're in this group because they're relatively calorie dense, which makes them undeniably satisfying even when eaten sparingly. So though I encourage you to use them for both snacks and cooking, you'll need to moderate their intake. Some tips: pre-portion a handful—rather than the whole bag—to bring with you to work, and always try to eat them in conjunction with Unlimited Foods.

They're so similar and interchangeable that all you need here are general guidelines: Choose whole, skin-on (unpeeled) nuts and seeds whenever possible. Like whole grains they're more nutritious and richer tasting; pre-chopped nuts go rancid more quickly. Store all nuts and seeds in the fridge or freezer to prolong their freshness, then just take out small quantities as you need them. Nuts find their way into all kinds of recipes in this book, from salads and soups to stir-fries and butters. Check out the Index for a full listing of where to find them.

VEGETABLE PROTEINS

This category of Flexible Foods includes non-dairy milks, tofus, tempeh, and seitan: one-time "hippie foods" that are now undeniably mainstream. It's important to note that all of these should be considered processed, if minimally so—that is, no more heavily manufactured than simple cheeses.

By the way, other kinds of store-bought vegan "meats" aren't Flexible Foods; their daunting ingredient lists put them into the realm of junk. And I'm no fan of textured vegetable protein (TVP) or products made from it, either; it's just another highly processed food. There are too many delicious, versatile sources of real vegetable protein to enjoy.

FLEXIBLE VEGETABLE PROTEINS

GROUP	BEST TYPE	HOW TO STORE	BEST WAYS TO PREPARE
NON-DAIRY MILKS	There's a lot more information in the sidebar on page XXX. But in a nutshell: soy and rice are now universally available in both refrigerated and shelf-stable forms. Other types to try: almond, hazelnut, oat, multigrain, and hemp. Coconut milk comes canned in full and reduced-fat forms—both are fine to use in these recipes. Always make sure whatever you buy is unflavored and unsweetened.	If it came refrigerated, keep it that way; otherwise refrigerate after opening. It keeps longer than cow's milk; at least a week or as long as two.	Use as is in coffee or tea; over cold cereal; cooked with grains into porridge; in smoothies, dressings, and sauces; or for baking.
FIRM TOFU	The kind in bricks, usually packed in water. (See the recipe and sidebar on page 113 for more detail.)	Once opened, store in fresh water or an airtight container for up to several days. For longer storage, freeze it, which has the added benefit of changing its texture so you can literally squeeze the water out before cooking.	Any way you would cook and use meat: microwave, steam, sauté and stir-fry, braise, roast or bake, grill or broil. You can also puree it into dips or use as a binder for loaves and burgers.
SILKEN TOFU	As the name implies, this tofu has a smooth, silky texture. It comes in soft, firm, and extra-firm textures, all interchangeable in recipes. (See the recipe and sidebar on page 113 for more detail.)	Silken tofu in aseptic packaging will keep in the cupboard for months; refrigerate after opening.	Use as you would eggs or custard: whip, blend, whisk, or heat in hot or cold dishes. It's also great dropped by the spoonful into soups and stews. Or try it in tofu scrambles instead of firm tofu for a more delicate texture.
TEMPEH	Made from fermented soybeans (and sometimes grains) that are pressed into flat blocks and sold refrigerated. This high-protein food has a distinctive slightly sour taste with *umami*—or savory—flavor.	Keep refrigerated and use up until a week after its sell-by date; it freezes well if you want to keep extra handy.	I prefer using it as a seasoning with other ingredients, much as you would use bacon or other smoked meats. So crumble and brown it like ground meat either in the oven or on the stove; it's also good in soups and stews.

THE TREAT PANTRY

It might seem counterintuitive to detail the "treats" you'll start eating after 6 P.M., but the majority of them are nutritious, necessary foods, and that's worthy of discussion. Junk will be easier to avoid, or at least minimize, if you have a clear idea of the place it should or shouldn't have in your diet.

The arrival of dusk isn't a license to go crazy and concoct a meal of junk. A VB6 dinner is based on ingredients from the Unlimited Foods group, augmented with moderate amounts of those from the Flexible Foods group, and enhanced with a little something from the lists that follow. If you want to maximize weight loss, choose fewer foods from the last Treats chart on page 40—or skip treats altogether on most days.

It's also important to consider quality when you go for treats. Ideally the flavor will be true and complex, and you'll end up eating less. Buy the best meat, chocolate, and white bread you can find (and, of course, afford); bake a pie for your next dinner party and savor one small (but delicious) slice; share a bottle of good wine with someone. I can guarantee your experience will be more satisfying in every way when you go beyond mass-produced junk to true luxuries for your treats—and you're more likely to eat less of them.

Every once in a while I find myself with a food from the Treat column on my plate before 6 o'clock, and you probably will too. Your awareness of these situations will help you balance them with meals that focus even more acutely on foods from the Unlimited and Flexible Foods groups.

The ultimate idea is to embrace and master give-and-take, perhaps the most important lesson for sustaining VB6 over the long term. If you think you need more "rules"—at least at the beginning—then I recommend adhering strictly to the VB6 regimen, excluding treats until evening rolls around. (I did that, fanatically, when I really wanted to lose weight, and it worked.) As you develop new habits, you will naturally learn how to incorporate treats into your day without abandoning the precepts of VB6 entirely.

To help you organize the way you think about the foods in this group and how you incorporate and substitute them in your diet, I've put them in categories. The sections that follow start with animal foods and continue to things like sweets and alcohol (the stuff that feels most like "treats").

EGGS AND DAIRY

Eggs and Parmesan cheese are my desert-island foods. Since I've mostly given them up during the day, I incorporate them into dinner more often than I used to, which has its own rewards: They're easy to prepare, go great together, and are satisfying and intensely flavored enough to keep me from eating red meat frequently. Think about starting with a plate of vegetables, then adding some grated cheese or a fried egg: a perfect little dish, and totally satisfying.

If you can, buy eggs from a local source (even city folk are keeping chickens these days).

Otherwise, read the label for descriptions about how the chickens were raised and what they were fed. Ditto with dairy. With the exception of the great cheeses, most dairy will be noticeably more tasty if it doesn't have to travel too far to get to you. Cheeses can be made from cow, sheep, or goat milk (or a combination); see the categories that follow to help you select and cook with them. And in all cases I prefer full-fat dairy to anything with reduced fat. The flavor is so much better and you're not eating that much of it.

TREAT EGGS AND DAIRY

PROTEIN GROUP	WHAT THEY ARE	HOW TO STORE	BEST WAYS TO PREPARE
EGGS	The labels are notoriously misleading and confusing, especially on mass-produced eggs. So look for words like "certified organic," "certified humane," "free farmed"; these distinctions give some indication that the chickens laying the eggs were raised better than conventional birds.	Eggs should always be kept in a cold part of the fridge (not the door); they should keep for as long as four to five weeks beyond the pack date or at least a week past their sell-by date. Eggs start to get noticeably watery when they're old.	There's no bad way to cook them: fried, scrambled, poached, hard- or soft-boiled in the shell, or baked. They're also a nice way to enrich pastas, soups, or stir-fries: Just beat, add, and stir.
HARD CHEESES	As cheese ages it loses moisture, so the texture becomes pleasantly gritty and crumbly and the flavor intensifies. This group includes Parmesan, Pecorino Romano, Manchego, Grana Padano, ricotta salata, Cotija, some goat cheeses, and others.	Store in parchment or wax paper and then in plastic or an airtight container; as long as they're kept free from moisture and air, they can last for weeks if not months in the fridge. If you happen to get a spot of mold on the outside, just cut it off; the cheese is still good.	These melt best when finely grated (a Microplane is perfect here); then add a sprinkling to eggs, stir-fries, soups, pastas, stews, gratins and casseroles, or sauces. Otherwise, grate or crumble them or shave slices with a vegetable peeler and add to salads, sandwiches, pesto, dips, or dressings.
SEMI-HARD AND SEMI-SOFT CHEESES	In general these aren't aged as long as the group above, and in fact some aren't aged at all. They range from the relatively soft, crumbly, veined blue cheeses like Gorgonzola, Roquefort, and other blues to rind cheeses like Brie and Camembert. Most Cheddars, some Mexican cheeses like Oaxacan, the Swiss cheeses, Monterey Jack, feta, and aged mozzarella and goat cheeses all fall into this group.	They don't last quite as long as hard cheeses; store (and trim off bad spots) the same way.	Most are good for slicing; the ones that aren't can be either grated or crumbled. Unlike hard cheeses, they melt well so they're good for both cooking and using raw for garnishing.

(continues)

PROTEIN GROUP	WHAT THEY ARE	HOW TO STORE	BEST WAYS TO PREPARE
SOFT CHEESES	The milky, tangy-tasting fresh cheeses. With the notable exception of fresh mozzarella, most are spreadable. Some others are ricotta, mascarpone, cream cheese, cottage cheese, fresh goat cheeses, quark.	Store in airtight containers and use within a week or two. (The really fresh ones should be eaten quickly.) Once they get moldy, they're no longer any good.	Spread or slice these cheeses atop salads, sandwiches, soups, pastas, stews, or casseroles, or stir into sauces or dips. Heat them gently if at all; some melt, while others dissolve and often curdle.
MILK	You can use milk with any fat percentage you like, though I prefer—and recommend—whole milk.	Refrigerate and stop using when it smells bad or curdles, usually a few days after its sell-by date.	Use milk for baking, making sauces and custards, marinating, or even poaching and baking.
BUTTER	Butter is just fat and a little water so it has almost the same calorie density as oil. Always buy unsalted butter (also called sweet butter) for a truer dairy flavor.	Store tightly wrapped in the refrigerator or freezer.	Use for baking, sautéing, pan roasting, or pan-frying—whenever you would use oil—but remember it burns at a lower temperature. A good strategy is to cut it half and half with olive or other oil so you get the flavor but can crank up the heat a little more.
CREAM	You want heavy—not whipping—cream, without any additives or emulsifiers. Avoid the stuff that's called "ultra-pasteurized"; it's ultra flavorless.	Keep cream in the coldest part of the fridge; it will last several days after its sell-by date.	Stir cream into soups, stews, sauces, or dressings for a silky, rich texture and a mild but milky flavor. Or whip it to serve with fruit.
SOUR CREAM	Sour cream is cream cultured with lactic acid bacteria, which makes it thick and tangy flavor. I use only full-fat sour cream.	Sour cream keeps for longer than other liquid dairy products but you store it the same way.	Add it to other ingredients over low heat, or use it as a last-minute garnish. If you heat it even to a simmer, it can curdle.
YOGURT	Yogurt is cultured milk. Look for "live, active cultures" and avoid yogurts with gelatins, gums, or stabilizers. The Greek-style yogurts are a good choice: thick and rich and everywhere now. I prefer full-fat but use whatever you like. Always choose unsweetened plain yogurts; forget the sugary stuff; sweeten your own with jam or honey if you like.	Yogurt keeps longer than other liquid dairy products, but you store it the same way. It usually keeps quite well past the expiration date.	Cooks and garnishes like sour cream; bakes like buttermilk; eats like ice cream (though usually needs a little sweetener!).

PROTEIN GROUP	WHAT THEY ARE	HOW TO STORE	BEST WAYS TO PREPARE
BUTTERMILK	True buttermilk is the liquid left behind after making butter. You can still find it in some farmers' markets and specialty stores. Otherwise what you get is essentially a thinned yogurt—a milk cultured with lactic acid bacteria.	Store in the coldest part of the refrigerator and use within a few days after the sell-by date.	Buttermilk promotes a tender crumb in biscuits and cakes. It's also good in cold sauces, dips, or dressings. To substitute for it in recipes, add 2 tablespoons white vinegar to 1¾ cup milk and let sit until it clots and thickens, about 10 minutes.
CRÈME FRAÎCHE	A thickened fresh cream that ranges from almost pourable to the consistency of commercial sour cream. It's got a slightly sweet, nutty taste.	Store in the coldest part of the refrigerator and use by the time it expires, or within a few days after the sell-by date.	Use crème fraîche to thicken dressings, sauces, or dips; or add it to enrich soups or stews (you can heat it almost to boiling without curdling). It's a good substitute for whipped cream as a topping or garnish.
ICE CREAM	Like milk it's made with varying percentages of fat. Go for the best you can find and buy it in small quantities. (Or make it yourself.)	It keeps for months in the freezer but the quality diminishes rapidly so eat it within a few days.	Lots of fruit with a little ice cream is an amazingly satisfying dessert.

FISH, POULTRY, AND MEAT

Raising and processing animals for food is among our most environmentally destructive activities. And eating high on the food chain generally doesn't do our bodies many favors either. So reducing your consumption is doubly beneficial and qualifies all fish, poultry, and meat as treats.

I'm not saying that these foods can't be included in a healthy diet; they can. But often the tendency is to eat them at the expense—or in some cases the exclusion—of plant foods. And when you consume less of them, you can usually buy better quality from sources that are more sustainable, less factorylike. This is also the best way to avoid meat, poultry, or fish that has been treated with hormones and antibiotics.

Eating seafood presents its own set of challenges. It is increasingly likely to be contaminated with pollutants and toxins; raising fish on farms can be especially tough on the environment; and many wild species have been overfished to near extinction. It takes a certain amount of homework to choose fish and shellfish that are sustainable and safe. There are several reliable sources to help consumers keep up with the latest information, but I always recommend The Monterey Bay Aquarium's Seafood Watch program: www.montereybayaquarium.org/cr/seafoodwatch.aspx. The comprehensive listings are updated constantly and easy to navigate.

Meat, poultry, and even fish are more interchangeable than you might realize. So if you want to make Chicken Stir-Fry in Lettuce Cups (page 172) but have only beef or pork, use one of them. Generally, try to replace like with like—lean cuts for lean, for example—but even that isn't a hard-and-fast rule since you can easily adjust the heat and cooking time to accommodate most change. The variations and ideas that follow the recipes will help you get started, and experience will build confidence. I'm confident as you experiment you'll come up with new ways to keep your diet fresh and lively. And that will make eating VB6 easy to sustain.

TREAT FISH, POULTRY, AND MEAT

PROTEIN GROUP	WHAT TO LOOK FOR	HOW TO STORE	BEST WAYS TO PREPARE
FISH	Wild-caught, sustainable species should always be your first choice. There are some farmed fish that are raised with minimal impact to their surrounding environment (like striped bass or catfish, but not salmon). Frozen fish is often a good option, as long as it's from a sustainable, safe source.	Keep packed in ice or stored in the coldest part of the refrigerator.	For cooking divide them into four categories: thin fillets (which are delicate), thick fillets (which are fairly sturdy), steaks (which are even sturdier), and whole fish. All can be poached, sautéed, pan- or deep-fried, or broiled. The sturdiest (and whole fish) can be roasted, braised, or grilled; timing depends on how thick they are and how high the heat is. Check fish frequently and you'll be fine: The second they turn opaque they're done.
SHELLFISH	A group that includes shrimp, clams, mussels, oysters, lobster, crab, crawfish, squid, octopus, and the like. Unless you live by a local source buy shrimp, squid, and crawfish frozen. Everything else should either be live or extremely fresh.	Keep packed in ice or stored in the coldest part of the refrigerator.	It's easiest to cook them in their shells, quickly with relatively high heat. Squid is best cooked super-fast over high heat; just the opposite is true for octopus.
CHICKEN	Look for heritage, local, or organic chickens before going to "natural" or free range, often meaningless distinctions unless there's more detail on the label.	Don't bother to re-wrap whole birds or parts if they're sealed in airtight packaging. Store fresh chicken in the refrigerator and eat it within a day or two, or freeze for up to a couple months.	Chicken can be cooked every way but generally the quickest are best: sautéed or stir-fried, grilled, or broiled. Bone-in pieces and whole birds are great—and super-easy to roast or braise.

PROTEIN GROUP	WHAT TO LOOK FOR	HOW TO STORE	BEST WAYS TO PREPARE
TURKEY, DUCK, AND GOOSE	The same labeling standards for chicken (or lack of them) apply to turkey. Avoid "self-basting" birds. Buy fresh when you can. Parts are undeniably convenient, especially if you're not going to eat that much in one sitting.	Store whole birds and parts the same way you would chicken.	It's now quite common to see these birds cut up into parts; turkey thighs are a great cut, especially braised. And like chicken, whole birds are easy to roast.
BEEF (AND VEAL)	"Natural" doesn't necessarily mean that the animals have been raised humanely, or even that they're free of hormones and antibiotics. Look for more specific information or buy from someone who can answer your questions.	If you buy big pieces, divide it into smaller cuts, wrap them tightly, and freeze them for another time. Store what you plan to use in the coldest part of the refrigerator and cook it within a day or two.	Cook beef any number of ways: stir-fried, grilled or broiled, roasted, pan-seared, or braised. Veal is the leaner, more tender alternative to beef, so it tends to get tough if you overcook it. And it's easier than you think to grind your own beef (or other meats) in the food processor; give it a try sometime.
PORK	The same label-reading advice for beef applies here, and then some. Industrially raised pork is barely worth eating. Well-raised pork is fatty and delicious; you don't need much of it to be satisfied.	Same as above: If you buy big pieces, divide into smaller cuts, wrap them tightly, and freeze them for another time. Store what you plan to use in the coldest part of the refrigerator and cook it within a day or two.	Pork is the most popular meat in the world for good reason: it's forgiving, takes to many seasoning profiles, and a little goes a long way. (Don't forget: bacon and sausage are usually pork.) Cook it the same way you would beef (see above).
LAMB	Americans hardly eat any lamb, which is a shame because it's so good and so easy to cook. Buy it the same way you do beef and pork. If you're lucky enough to have a good local source, use it.	Divide it up and freeze what you don't need for another time. Store what you plan to use in the refrigerator and cook it within a day.	Lamb can also impart huge amounts of flavor with small quantities. Cook it on the grill, roasted, pan-seared, braised, stewed, or stir-fried.
SMOKED AND CURED MEATS	The most bang for your buck, since with VB6 you truly use them as seasoning. Bacon, smoked sausages (which are more intensely flavored than fresh; my favorite is chorizo), salamis, hams (including Prosciutto and Serrano), and specialty cuts like pancetta and guanicale.	Curing and smoking are ways of preserving meat, so most of the foods in this category will keep for weeks—if not months—in the refrigerator. Another reason to have at least one handy at all times.	Think of smoked and cured meats as seasonings. Chop them up and sauté them before adding vegetables to the pan, use them as the foundation for soups and sauces, toss a little into a pot of beans.

THE "TREAT" TREATS—AND JUNK

Though I discourage dubbing foods either "good" or "bad," VB6 places everything on a continuum. And here are the ultimate treats on that spectrum: the stuff that has the most sugar and refined carbohydrates and the lowest nutritional value. They're presented loosely in order of how prevalent they are in my diet—again with the reasoning that even if this section might state the obvious, mindfulness is the key to successful VB6 living.

I love crusty French baguettes, but I don't eat them every day; the same goes for chocolate or sweetened condiments. That is, after all, why they're called treats.

TREAT GROUP	WHAT THEY ARE	HOW TO STORE	BEST WAYS TO USE
WHITE FLOUR, PASTA, RICE, AND NOODLES	These are all the more processed version of their brown counterparts (the semolina in pasta could be considered slightly less processed than white flour), with the fiber and many nutrients stripped away. It might sound impossible now, but once you start eating less of them these foods will come to feel like indulgences. Nice indulgences.	Store starches in airtight containers in the pantry. Wrap raw doughs tightly and freeze for up to a couple months; then thaw in the refrigerator before using. Even bread freezes well if wrapped tightly. See the sidebar on page 251 for some ideas on what to do with bits and pieces of leftover loaves.	Some tips: Avoid bleached white flour entirely, and try cutting recipes that use white flour with up to half whole wheat flour. The best white rice is short grain (for risottos and paellas) or basmati or jasmine (for steaming and pilafs). And the best dried pastas usually come from Italy (if you have access to great fresh pasta, go for it). Try changing the proportion of these "white" ingredients in recipes to emphasize the vegetables instead.
DRIED FRUIT	Raisins, cranberries, apricots, pineapple, dates, figs—any fruit that's been dehydrated. The reason fresh and frozen fruit is unlimited and dried fruit is a treat is that the concentration of sugar in dried is so high (and water content so low).	Keep in an airtight container in the pantry. Most dried fruits will keep for several months.	Use dried fruit as a garnish or sweetener—in dishes like pilafs or salads—and keep the fresh or frozen fruit around for snack time.
DARK CHOCOLATE	For the most flavor and nutrients—and less sugar and fillers—the darker the better. Look for chocolate with 60 percent or higher cocoa content (the better ones are labeled that way). If you're a devout milk or white chocolate eater, that's okay, but know that dark chocolate is lower on the treat-o-meter.	Store chocolate in a dark space at room temperature. It will keep for 1 to 2 years.	Whether you eat great dark chocolate out of hand, stir it into cookie dough, or melt it into sauce, there are few more satisfying indulgences. Enjoy it, and avoid the junk.

TREAT GROUP	WHAT THEY ARE	HOW TO STORE	BEST WAYS TO USE
SWEETENERS	Sugars, syrups, and the like. I don't see all the fuss about agave nectar, but you can use it if you like; honey, strictly speaking, isn't vegan but except for the most commercial brands it's as good and natural a sweetener as there is (real maple syrup is also terrific). Plain table sugar also falls into this category.	None of these sweeteners needs to be refrigerated; keep them in a container in the pantry. (You'll be amazed how slowly you go through them.)	The perception of sweetness varies among individuals and will likely change as you eat less of it. Try to rely on fruit whenever possible in baked foods and desserts. Second choice: Use raw turbinado sugar, honey, or maple syrup; at least you'll get some flavor in the bargain. If you're using sugar to balance acidity in savory dishes, a pinch isn't going to hurt (unless you're diabetic).
SWEETENED CONDIMENTS	You know them: ketchup, relish, barbecue sauce, fruit syrups, caramel; or sweet glazes, marinades, dressings, or sauces.	Refrigerate once open, if necessary, and follow expiration dates.	Try making your own, especially dressing; once you remove the sugar and unrecognizable additives it becomes a Flexible Food. If you must buy bottled stuff, do your best to avoid prepared condiments with high fructose corn syrup. You'll be shocked to see how much sugar (and chemicals) they can pack into 1 tablespoon of liquid; so pourer beware.
ALCOHOL	Beer, wine, liquor, spirits—all booze.	Store alcohol in a dark, cool space. Shelf life depends on the type and vintage of the alcohol. Most beer and white and rosé wines are best served chilled.	Choosing if to drink, when to drink, and how much is a personal decision. Just be aware that alcohol sits right below white bread and just a tad above sodas when it comes to nutrition, providing carbohydrates that quickly break down into sugars. But there is also evidence that if consumed in moderation, alcohol can have several health benefits, along with the obvious calming effect. In that way, if you're going to drink, it makes sense to think of it as any other VB6 treat.
ANYTHING HIGHLY PROCESSED	Junk, in other words. You know it when you see it.	Most of it is meant for immediate consumption, but some things like chips and crackers keep extremely well so if you're concerned about your willpower, keep them out of sight. Out of the house, in fact.	There is no real use for these foods other than sensory gratification, though I'm human and I recognize they're ubiquitous and virtually unavoidable. At every turn, look for other choices first.

A MONTH OF VB6

Use this 28-day menu any way you'd like: You can follow it verbatim, you can dip in and out of it whenever you need inspiration, or you might breeze through to get an idea of what a day of eating VB6 looks like. It's also a handy, at-a-glance way to preview many of the recipes and variations in the book.

WEEK 1

	BREAKFAST	LUNCH	SNACK	DINNER	DESSERT
DAY 1	Green Apple Stir-Fry with Cashews (page 76)	Eggplant Meatballs (page 124) + Everyday Salad Bowl (page 224)	Lime Tortilla Crisps (page 137)	Red Paella with Scallops (page 167) + cooked kale (page 227)	Avocado Chocolate Mousse with Raspberries (page 211)
DAY 2	Strawberry Balsamic Smoothie (page 48)	Escarole and White Bean Soup (page 107) + Breadsticks (page 250)	Korean-Style Cucumber Quickles (page 138)	Risotto with Charred Brussels Sprouts (page 159) cooked carrots (page 227)	Pears with Crisp Topping (page 212)
DAY 3	Green Toast (page 55)	Chickpea Tabbouleh (page 96) + Everyday Salad Bowl (page 224)	Raspberry Sorbet on a Stick (page 152)	Jerk Chicken Burgers (page 178) + cooked broccoli (page 227)	Coconut Brown Rice Pudding with Pineapple (page 219)
DAY 4	No-Bake Pumpkin Custard (page 79)	Chopped Salad with Tahini Dressing (page 92) + cooked beans (page 232)	Miso Jerky (page 148)	Sausage Hash (page 190) + Everyday Salad Bowl (page 224)	Peanut Butter Bonbons (page 210)
DAY 5	Broccoli Scramble (page 72)	Grains Marinara (page 108) + Everyday Salad Bowl (page 224)	Wasabimame (page 135)	Mussels, Corn, and Noodles in Coconut Broth (page 170)	Summer Pudding with Vanilla Cream (page 207)
DAY 6	Lime-Mango Parfait (page 53)	Teriyaki Tempeh with Bok Choy (page 122)	Radishes with Avocado Dip (page 147)	Pumpkin Pasta (page 157) + Everyday Salad Bowl (page 224)	Port-Marinated Figs (page 206)
DAY 7	"Chorizo" Tacos (page 81)	Soba with Summer Squash, Mushrooms, and Sea Greens (page 111)	Banana-Peanut Truffles (page 151)	African-Style Chicken Stew (page 180) + wheat berries (page 230)	Banana-Chocolate Ice Cream (page 208)

WEEK 2

	BREAKFAST	LUNCH	SNACK	DINNER	DESSERT
DAY 8	Walnut Banana Bread (page 86)	Curried Spinach and Tofu (page 119)	Jícama with Jalapeño "Mayo" (page 142)	Schezuan Beef and Celery (page 194) + cooked quinoa (page 230)	Gingery Mango Pudding (page 205)
DAY 9	Beans on Toast (page 59)	Caponata Mixed Rice (page 114) + Everyday Salad Bowl (page 224)	Chile-Cherry Gorpcorn (page 133)	Vegetable Curry with Lamb (page 200) + VB6 Bread, Six Ways (page 249)	Decadent Oatmeal Cookies (page 214)
DAY 10	Blueberry Oatmeal Pancakes (page 84)	Fully Loaded Black Bean Burritos (page 117)	Endive with Mushroom-Olive Tapenade (page 140)	Turkey Shepherd's Pie (page 191) + Everyday Salad Bowl (page 224)	Cherry Clafoutis (page 217)
DAY 11	Super Vegetable Porridge (page 70)	Hearty Miso Soup (page 101)	Fruit Candy (page 150)	Steak au Poivre with Mushrooms (page 197) + boiled new potatoes	Grapefruit with Spiced Crisp Topping (page 212)
DAY 12	Morning Milkshake (page 52)	Mushroom-Nut Burgers over Greens (page 129)	Southwestern Bean Dip with Peppers (page 144)	Chicken with Fennel Salad (page 175) + brown rice (page 230)	Rice Pudding with Slow-Roasted Fruit (page 218)
DAY 13	Muesli (page 62)	Tofu Tomato Sauce over Spaghetti (page 110)	Melon-Cucumber on a Stick (page 152)	Pane Cotto (page 161) + cooked spinach (page 227)	Balsamic Strawberries with Black Pepper and Ricotta (page 206)
DAY 14	Plum Jam on Toast (page 58)	Rhubarb and Red Lentil Soup (page 103) + Breadsticks (page 250)	Salt and Vinegar Chickpeas (page 136)	Jícama Salad with Salmon Steaks (page 163) + quinoa (page 230)	Chocolate Almond Avocado Mousse (page 211)

WEEK 3

	BREAKFAST	LUNCH	SNACK	DINNER	DESSERT
DAY 15	Spiced Bulgur Pilaf (page 65)	Creamy Tomato Soup (page 106) + Breadsticks (page 250)	Cucumbers with Miso-Carrot Dipping Sauce (page 141)	Pork Chop Pan Roast (page 188) + Everyday Salad Bowl (page 224)	Banana-Mango Ice Cream (page 208)
DAY 16	Gingery Kale Smoothie (page 51)	Edamame Fried Rice (page 115)	Japanese-Style Mushroom Quickles (page 138)	Chicken Stir-Fry in Lettuce Cups (page 172) + brown rice (page 230)	Grown-Up Summer Pudding (page 207)
DAY 17	Coco-Oat-Nut Granola (page 62)	Tofu Ceviche (page 94) + Everyday Salad Bowl (page 224)	Rosemary–White Bean Dip with Fennel (page 144)	Pork, Asparagus, and Soba (page 185)	Apples with Crisp Maple Topping (page 212)
DAY 18	Pita Pizza with Fresh Jam (page 56)	Slow-Cooked Brussels Sprouts with Lemongrass (page 121)	Garlicky Tofu Jerky (page 148)	Open-Face Bánh Mì Sandwiches (page 193) + cooked cauliflower (page 227)	Banana Cream Pie Ice Cream (page 208)
DAY 19	Salsa Sweet Potato (page 74)	Peas and Carrots Salad (page 97) + Everyday Salad Bowl (page 224)	Tropical Gorpcorn (page 134)	Stir-Fried White Beans and Shrimp with Fennel (page 169) + whole wheat spaghetti	Gingered Apricot Clafoutis (page 217)
DAY 20	Cornmeal Mush with Many Toppings (page 67)	Cold Sesame Noodles with Crisp Tofu Cubes (page 112)	Curried Mango Dip (page 147)	Gingered Rice with Chicken (page 176)	Thick and Cold Rice Pudding (page 219)
DAY 21	Scrambled Sweet and Hot Peppers (page 71)	Vegetable Pot Pie (page 123)	Srirachamame (page 135)	Gingery Winter Stew (page 183) + Everyday Salad Bowl (page 224)	Mexican Chocolate Avocado Mousse (page 211)

WEEK 4

	BREAKFAST	LUNCH	SNACK	DINNER	DESSERT
DAY 22	Almond Quinoa (page 68)	Cauliflower Romesco Soup (page 118) + Breadsticks (page 250)	Spanish-Style Chickpea Dip with Carrots (page 144)	Tuscan Chicken Stew (page 182) + Everyday Salad Bowl (page 224)	Vegan (or Not) Chocolate Chunk Oatmeal Cookies (page 214)
DAY 23	Sweet Red Bean Breakfast (page 78)	Moroccan Potato Salad (page 98) + Everyday Salad Bowl (page 224)	Basil Gorpcorn (page 134)	Grits and Portabello Grillades (page 199) + cooked broccoli (page 227)	Banana-Chocolate-Hazelnut Ice Cream (page 208)
DAY 24	Blueberry Spoonbread (page 69)	Fava Bean Salad (page 93) + Everyday Salad Bowl (page 224)	Garlic Tortillas (page 137)	Chicken Vegetable Tagine (page 179)	Boozy Pineapple with Maple Yogurt (page 206)
DAY 25	P.B. & J. Couscous (page 63)	Curried Carrot and Lentil Soup (page 102) + Breadsticks (page 250)	Wasabi Peas (page 135)	Crisp Pork on Green Papaya Salad (page 187) + wheat berries (page 230)	Peanut Butter Truffles (page 210)
DAY 26	Berry Smoothie (page 50)	Curried Spinach with Tomatoes and Chickpeas (page 119)	French-Style Radish Quickles (page 138)	Chicken Burgers with Vietnamese Flavors (page 178) + Everyday Salad Bowl (page 224)	Tropical Fruit Pudding (page 205)
DAY 27	Grain Nuts with Fruit (page 61)	E.L.T. Sandwich (page 126) + Everyday Salad Bowl (page 224)	Mushroom-Green Olive Tapenade (page 140)	Fish with Vegetable Gratin (page 164)	Blueberry-Lemon Clafoutis (page 217)
DAY 28	Apple-Oat Muffins (page 85)	Ribollita (page 99) + Breadsticks (page 250)	Frozen Tropical Truffles (page 151)	Beef Stew with Pistachios, Beets, and Greens (page 180) + brown rice (page 230)	Chocolate-Cherry-Coconut Pudding (page 205)

BREAKFAST

CHERRY VANILLA SMOOTHIE

BERRY SMOOTHIE

GINGERY KALE SMOOTHIE

MORNING MILKSHAKE

ORANGE-PEACH PARFAIT

GREEN TOAST

PITA PIZZA WITH FRESH JAM

FRESH BLACKBERRY JAM
ON TOAST

BEANS ON TOAST

GRAIN NUTS WITH FRUIT

COCO-OAT-NUT GRANOLA

P.B. & J. COUSCOUS

WALK-AWAY OATMEAL

SPICED BULGUR PILAF

CORNMEAL MUSH WITH
MANY TOPPINGS

ALMOND QUINOA

BLUEBERRY SPOONBREAD

VB6 JOOK

SCRAMBLED SWEET AND HOT
PEPPERS

BROCCOLI SCRAMBLE

GOOD MORNING SWEET POTATO

GREEN APPLE STIR-FRY WITH
CASHEWS

SWEET RED BEAN BREAKFAST

NO-BAKE PUMPKIN CUSTARD

"CHORIZO" TACOS

CRISP QUINOA-CORN CAKES

COCONUT HOECAKES WITH
MANGO SALSA

BLUEBERRY OATMEAL PANCAKES

APPLE-OAT MUFFINS

WALNUT BANANA BREAD

Morning in America is typically anything but vegan, and many people find breakfast is the hardest meal of the day to change. It was for me, and sometimes still is, which is why I give in once in a while and have sausage, bacon, or eggs. (But just once in a while, and on those days I eat vegan the rest of the day.)

The key is to try: This chapter delivers a wide variety of delicious, high-fiber, protein-rich foods that fill you up and keep you satisfied through the long haul to lunch. If you're reluctant, get ready to be surprised: I'm confident that if you are willing to "practice," you'll come to find eating this way not only enjoyable but also convenient.

Many of the recipes here—toasted bread, smoothies, and baked treats—will be familiar. Others are quick to assemble from pre-cooked grains and make-ahead components like nut butters and fresh fruit jams. Some, like stuffed sweet potatoes or baked oatmeal, can be popped in the microwave or oven while you get ready for the day. Can't imagine having time to prepare anything before you head out the door? Fine, take an apple muffin with you or stock your office with cold cereal, non-dairy milk, and fruit—*always* lots of fruit.

On the weekends, when there's time to do more cooking, tofu scrambles and griddle cakes are utterly brunch-worthy. And if you're like me, you'll stop craving sweets in the morning and gravitate toward savory leftovers from last night's dinner. With that mindset, almost everything in the fridge suddenly qualifies as breakfast.

The important thing to remember, though, is that this is a lifestyle, not a rulebook. As I said: Once in a blue moon I revert to my non-vegan ways and scramble up a batch of eggs. Everyone deserves a treat once in a while.

CHERRY VANILLA SMOOTHIE

MAKES 1 serving   **TIME** 5 minutes

This is so indulgent it will remind you of old-fashioned ice cream. And since smoothies are easy to vary depending on what you have and what you like, use this recipe to play; the variations will help get you started.

½ cup unsweetened plain non-dairy milk or silken tofu (4 ounces)

½ teaspoon vanilla extract

1 cup fresh or unsweetened frozen pitted cherries, or a little more

Ice as needed

1   Put the ingredients into a blender in the order listed, adding ice only if using fresh fruit; if you're using frozen fruit you probably won't need any ice.

2   Puree until smooth, stopping the machine once or twice to scrape down the sides. Adjust the texture with a little water or ice, or more cherries. Serve immediately.

VARIATIONS

STRAWBERRY BALSAMIC SMOOTHIE Swap 1 teaspoon balsamic vinegar for the vanilla and strawberries for the cherries.

MELON LIME SMOOTHIE Swap 1 tablespoon fresh lime juice for vanilla and cubed melon for the cherries. Great made with a little coconut milk (reduced-fat is fine) in place of half of the non-dairy milk. Add a pinch dried or fresh chile, if you like.

AVOCADO BANANA SMOOTHIE Swap ½ avocado and ½ frozen banana for the cherries; you'll almost certainly need more ice.

MORE IDEAS

Vary the seasonings and flavorings with fresh herbs like basil or mint or spices like cinnamon, nutmeg, or cardamom.

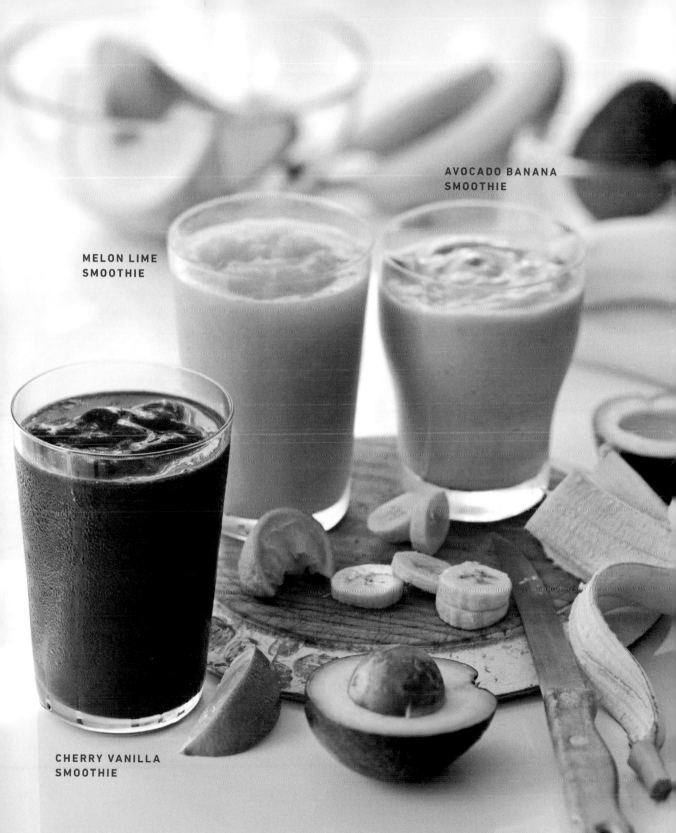

AVOCADO BANANA
SMOOTHIE

MELON LIME
SMOOTHIE

CHERRY VANILLA
SMOOTHIE

BERRY SMOOTHIE

MAKES 1 serving   TIME 5 minutes

A perfect VB6 breakfast: fast, portable, satisfying, and tasty. It is easily
varied, and can taste different each time you make it, depending on
which type of milk you use. Without the tang of yogurt, you won't need
any added sugar, but if you want to re-create some of that creamy texture,
substitute silken tofu for the non-dairy milk. Store-bought frozen
fruit—not only berries, but also mangos, peaches, and so on (see the list
below)—is more convenient and often even tastier.

½ cup unsweetened
non-dairy milk or silken
tofu (4 ounces)

½ fresh or frozen banana,
cut into chunks

1 cup fresh or unsweetened
frozen strawberries, or a
little more

Ice as needed

1   Put the first three ingredients into a blender in the order listed,
adding ice only if using fresh fruit; if you're using frozen fruit, you
probably won't need any ice.

2   Puree until smooth, stopping the machine once or twice to scrape
down the sides. Adjust the texture to be as thin or thick as you like with
a little water or ice, or more berries. Serve immediately.

MORE IDEAS

Use blueberries, blackberries, boysenberries, or pitted cherries, alone
or in combination. • Fresh peaches or apricots are a seasonal treat; don't
bother to peel them. (Frozen are fine, too.) • Melons make terrific smoothies, especially cantaloupe and honeydew. • Cut-up tropical fruit is good:
Mangos or papaya make super-rich smoothies; pineapples are good and tart.
• A few tomatoes, alone or in combination with other fruit, can be shockingly
good. (Again, no need to remove the peels.) Try them sometime. • Season the
smoothie with lemon or lime juice, vanilla, or even a pinch of ground hot red
chile or salt and pepper.

MAN VS. MACHINE

To make sure all your smoothies turn smooth in the blender, put
the ingredients in the machine in this order: liquid, fruit (frozen or
fresh), then a few ice cubes if you're using fresh fruit. Start on a
low speed, gradually increasing once things start swirling. Add ice
or water—or more fruit—to get the thickness and heft you want.
Stop to scrape down the sides or stir the contents as necessary.
And, yes, for a single serving you can use a food processor without
overflowing the work bowl, but your smoothie won't be as smooth.

GINGERY KALE SMOOTHIE

MAKES 1 serving   TIME 10 minutes

Tal Ronen, the chef of LYFE Kitchen, turned me on to what just five years ago would have been an unthinkably bizarre smoothie. Yet it works; the flavor is slightly sweet and distinctively gingery, and it's as good before dinner as it is before dawn.

2 tablespoons fresh lemon juice

½ cup chopped cucumber

½ fresh or frozen banana

1 packed cup chopped kale leaves

½ inch ginger, peeled

1 apple, unpeeled, cut into chunks

½ cup ice, or more as needed

Seltzer or tap water as needed

1   Put the ingredients into a blender in the order listed with ½ cup of the ice and reserving the seltzer.

2   Puree until smooth, stopping to push the ingredients toward the blade; once the machine gets moving, stop once or twice more to scrape down the sides. Adjust the texture with more ice or a little seltzer. Serve immediately.

MORE IDEAS

In place of the banana, try pear or honeydew melon (1 cup chopped fruit).
• Spinach, watercress, or arugula can also be substituted for the kale.
• Increase the cucumber to 1¼ cups and skip the apple.

THE CASE FOR FROZEN BANANAS

Frozen bananas are amazing, especially when pureed or mashed with something else. They freeze—and unpeel—amazingly well, right in their skins; it's as if you're suspending their ripeness in time. Once reanimated, everything they touch becomes richer and creamier and their flavor is almost always overridden by other ingredients.

Store ripe bananas—unpeeled!—directly in the freezer. (Or if you don't want them just floating around in there, put them in an airtight bag or container so you can just pop them in and take them out at will.) The skins will turn solid black but the flesh inside will be perfectly fine until they get freezer burn; then it's time to say good-bye. But if you drink a couple smoothies every week, they probably won't sit around for long. Make the smoothies on pages 48, 50, and 51, and the Walnut Banana Bread on page 86. And try the bonbons and ice cream on pages 208 and 210.

MORNING MILKSHAKE

MAKES 1 serving   **TIME** 5 minutes

As smoothies go, this is a pretty decadent one, thus the name: perfect for
those with a morning sweet tooth.

¾ cup unsweetened plain
non-dairy milk

1 fresh or frozen banana,
cut into chunks

1 tablespoon unsweetened
cocoa

1 teaspoon sugar,
preferably turbinado

Ice as needed

1   Put the ingredients into a blender in the order listed; if you're using a
frozen banana you probably won't need much ice, so hold off at first.

2   Puree until smooth, stopping once or twice to scrape down the sides.
Adjust the texture with a little water or ice. Serve immediately.

MORE IDEAS

Make this smoothie more substantial by adding up to 2 tablespoons chopped
nuts. • Use coconut milk for up to ¼ cup of the liquid. Add 1 tablespoon
unsweetened shredded coconut if you'd like.

SAYING GOOD-BYE TO COW'S MILK

People tell me that giving up dairy in their morning coffee is
unthinkable. Being a half-and-half fan (who's also somewhat aller-
gic to dairy), I get it.

In fact, changing dietary habits is never easy. All I can do is
encourage you to try non-dairy milks or even nothing—always an
option—at least on most days. Then make a tablespoon or so of
cow's milk in the morning an occasional treat. If you're a cereal
eater or a by-the-glass or grande latte drinker, then it's even more
important you find a dairy substitute you like. (Having said all of
that, if a dash of half-and-half in your coffee is a cheat that will
help you be VB6 otherwise, that's not a bad trade-off.)

Ten years ago you'd have been hard pressed to find soy milk outside of a health food store. Now there are non-dairy milks extracted
from oats, rice, soy, hemp, mixed grains, and all kinds of nuts, to
be found in both the refrigerated case and the center aisles of most
supermarkets.

Use only those that are unflavored and unsweetened. Like cow's
and goat's milk, non-dairy milks contain a fair amount of natural
sugar (usually glucose), and I'm disappointed to report that additives like gums and vitamins are often added. This isn't terrible, but
it's also unnecessary; see the sidebar on page 61 to see how easily
vegan milk can be made at home.

ORANGE-PEACH PARFAIT

MAKES 4 servings   TIME 10 minutes

Dessert for breakfast—pretty enough for Sunday brunch, simple enough to layer in a jar and bring with you to work. Somewhat surprisingly, white balsamic vinegar helps bring out the sweetness of the peaches, but if you don't have any, just skip it; substituting another vinegar isn't the same.

4 peaches, sliced (or about 4 cups frozen)

1 tablespoon white balsamic vinegar (optional)

24 ounces silken tofu (about 3 cups)

2 tablespoons fresh orange juice

1 tablespoon maple syrup or other sweetener, or more to taste

2 teaspoons grated orange zest

½ teaspoon salt

1   Combine the peaches and the vinegar (if you're using it) in a medium bowl and stir to combine. Let sit on the counter, stirring occasionally, until the peaches release some juice, about 5 minutes.

2   Whisk together the tofu, orange juice, syrup, zest, and salt until smooth. (It will go through an awkward "broken" stage but just keep whisking until the mixture emulsifies.) Taste and adjust the seasoning or sweetness as you like.

3   Put some tofu mixture in the bottom of a large glass bowl (or tall glasses for individual servings). Top with some of the peaches and their juice, and repeat, alternating to build a layered parfait. Serve right away or cover and refrigerate for up to 1 hour or so.

VARIATIONS

LIME-MANGO PARFAIT Swap fresh lime juice and zest for the orange and mango for the peaches.

LEMON-BLUEBERRY PARFAIT Swap 1 tablespoon fresh lemon juice and 1 teaspoon zest for the orange and blueberries for the peaches.

BLACK PEPPER-STRAWBERRY PARFAIT A classic Italian combination that sounds wild but tastes great. Use dark balsamic vinegar instead of white and strawberries instead of peaches. Add several grinds of pepper to the mixture in Step 1. In the tofu preparation, substitute 1 tablespoon fresh lemon juice and 1 teaspoon lemon zest for the orange juice and zest.

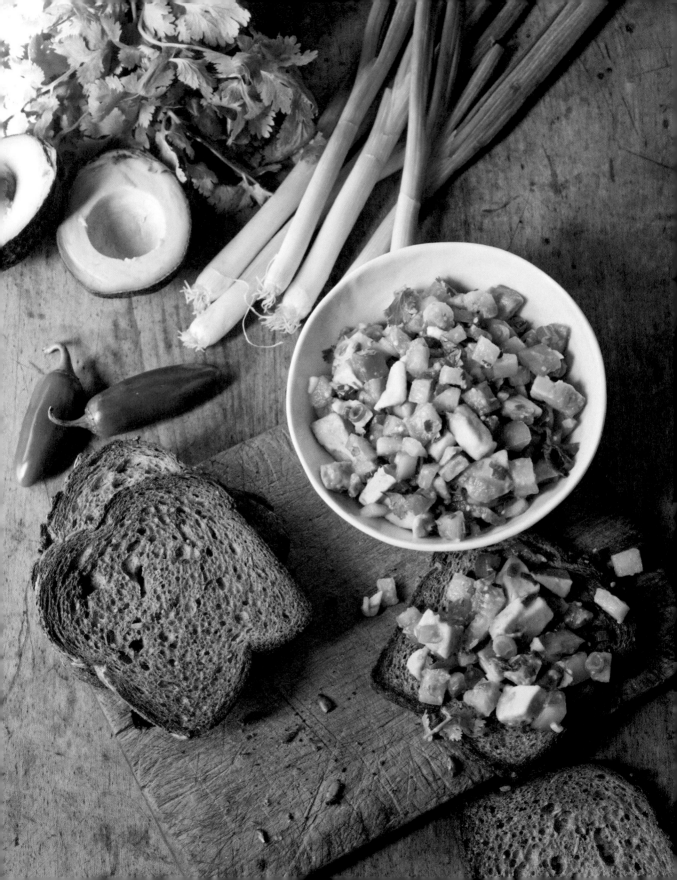

GREEN TOAST

MAKES 4 servings   **TIME** 15 minutes

Think of this as a gorgeous fruit salad that just happens to be green. And savory. You control how much heat you want, including skipping the chiles all together if you prefer. And this topping is also good—for breakfast or otherwise—tossed into rice or scooped up with baked plain corn tortillas.

1 pound tomatillos, chopped

2 avocados, chopped

2 scallions, chopped

1 or 2 fresh hot chiles
(like jalapeño or serrano),
seeded

1 teaspoon minced garlic

½ cup chopped fresh
cilantro

2 tablespoons fresh lime
juice, or more to taste

1 teaspoon salt

4 slices whole-grain toast

1   Put the tomatillos, avocados, scallions, chiles, garlic, cilantro, lime juice, and salt in a medium bowl.

2   Toss the mixture until just combined. Taste and adjust the seasoning, adding more lime juice if you'd like. Spoon over the toast and serve right away, or let it sit a few minutes so the bread soaks up the juices and softens.

MORE IDEAS

Try cantaloupe, honeydew, or casaba melon instead of the tomatillos.
• Use ripe tomatoes for some or all of the tomatillos.

PITA PIZZA WITH FRESH JAM

MAKES 4 servings   **TIME** About 30 minutes

Inspired by Pop-Tarts, the icon in a category of junky breakfasts known as "toaster pastries," here's an equivalent that is (obviously) better for you and almost as simple, especially if you use a toaster oven. In fact, once you prepare the fruit and buy the pita, you've got three breakfasts that are toaster-fast (see the variations). Your strawberries may be sweet enough that they don't even need sugar; taste one before you start to make the jam.

Four 8-inch pitas, preferably whole wheat

2 tablespoons olive oil

½ cup warm water

2 tablespoons sugar, preferably turbinado (optional)

2 cups strawberries or other berries, chopped

½ cup chopped pistachios

1 Heat the oven to 425°F. Brush the tops of the pitas with the oil and spread them out on a large baking sheet.

2 Put ½ cup water in a medium saucepan over medium-high heat and whisk in the sugar, if you're using it; bring to a boil. Stir in the strawberries and cook, mashing and stirring until the fruit softens, 2 or 3 minutes. Strain (reserving the liquid for another use if you'd like).

3 Spread the compote on the pitas and sprinkle with the pistachios; press the nuts down into the jam a bit so they don't burn.

4 Transfer the pizzas to the oven and bake until the pitas brown around the edges and the nuts turn golden, 5 to 10 minutes. Cut each pita into quarters and serve warm or at room temperature.

VARIATIONS

SAVORY BREAKFAST PIZZA Pitas are the perfect vehicle for cooked vegetables, especially grilled ones. Skip the fruit and sugar. Keep the pistachios or try other chopped nuts. Roughly mash soft cooked vegetables like eggplant, zucchini, greens, cauliflower, or mushrooms and spread them on the bread instead of the compote in Step 3; season with salt, pepper, and whatever herbs or spices you like.

TOASTER PITA TO GO Make the topping in advance and prepare the pitas one at a time as needed: cut the breads in half crosswise and toast them. Spread the jam inside the pocket (if there is one) or between the two pieces; sprinkle with the nuts and eat like a sandwich.

MORE IDEAS

Virtually any fruit works here, from plums and nectarines to all the other berries. Trim and peel them as needed, then chop them into small pieces before cooking. • Whole wheat lavash, naan, and chapati are all excellent substitutes for the pita. • And of course use whatever nuts you have and like. Seeds are good too, as is unsweetened shredded coconut.

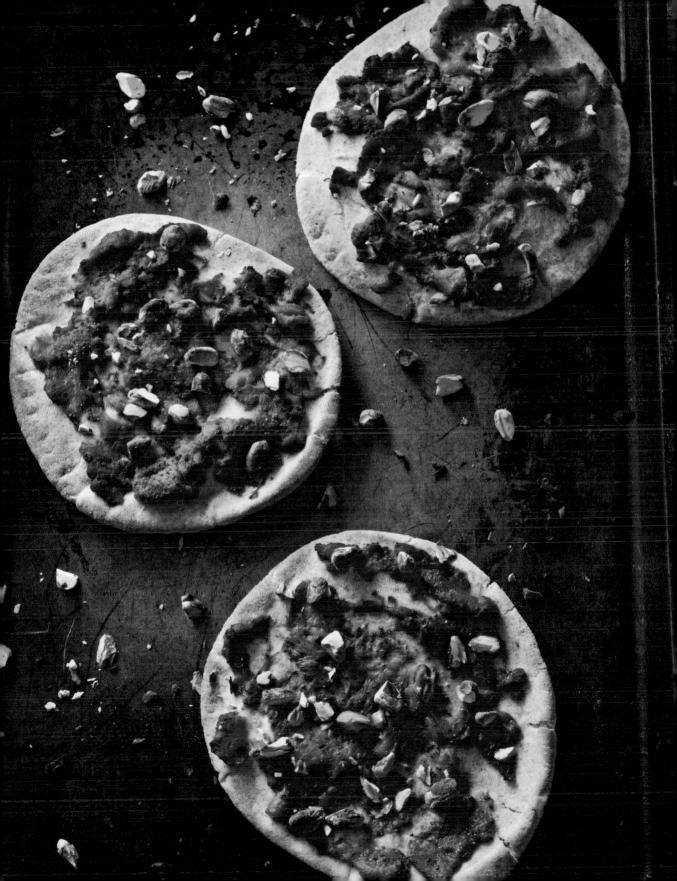

FRESH BLACKBERRY JAM ON TOAST

MAKES 4 servings (about 2 cups)   **TIME** About 45 minutes

Making jam at home from seasonal fruit, whether cooked or uncooked, is unbelievably simple and fast. It's a much healthier option and way more delicious than most store-bought jams, which often contain little or no fiber and loads of sugar. The difference is really night and day.

4 cups blackberries, rinsed

2 tablespoons maple syrup or other sweetener

¼ teaspoon ground cardamom, plus more to taste

¼ teaspoon salt

4 thick slices whole-grain toast

1 Put the berries in a broad shallow bowl, drizzle with the syrup, and sprinkle with the cardamom and salt. Mash the mixture with a fork or potato masher until the berries are a little broken up and thicken into a spreadable paste.

2 Taste and adjust the seasoning, adding more cardamom if you'd like. Spread on the toast (or transfer to a jar and refrigerate until you're ready to use. The jam will keep in the refrigerator for a few days.)

VARIATIONS

SPICED TOMATO JAM ON TOAST This you've got to cook, and it will keep for a week or so. Instead of the blackberries, use chopped ripe tomatoes or drain 2 cans diced tomatoes (reserve their juice if you'd like); add 1 minced jalapeño chile or a pinch of cayenne for a little heat. Bring to a boil in a medium saucepan over medium heat, stirring occasionally. Lower the heat to a bubble and cook, stirring occasionally, until the mixture darkens and thickens, 25 to 30 minutes.

PLUM JAM ON TOAST Substitute 1½ pounds plums for the blackberries; pit and chop them, then follow the cooking directions for the tomato jam variation above.

MORE IDEAS

Swap strawberries or raspberries for the blackberries. • Use cinnamon instead of cardamom. • Throw in ½ cup chopped fresh basil or mint.

BEANS ON TOAST

MAKES 4 servings   TIME 15 minutes

A traditional British breakfast, often eaten with a cup of hot tea. It's just as good with coffee, or over a cup of rice, grains, or cooked vegetables for that matter.

3 cups cooked or canned navy beans (see page 232)

2 tablespoons minced onion

2 tablespoons tomato paste

1 tablespoon maple syrup or other sweetener

1 tablespoon cider vinegar

1 teaspoon Dijon mustard, or more to taste

1 teaspoon soy sauce, or more to taste

4 slices whole-grain bread

1 Drain the beans. If you made them yourself, reserve the cooking liquid; if they're canned, discard the liquid and rinse the beans. Combine the beans, onion, tomato paste, syrup, vinegar, mustard, and soy sauce in a medium saucepan over medium heat.

2 Cook, stirring occasionally and adding water as necessary so that so that the mixture doesn't stick to the pan, until the onion softens and the beans are coated in a glossy sauce, 5 to 10 minutes.

3 Meanwhile, toast the bread. Taste the beans and adjust the seasonings, adding more soy sauce or mustard if you like. Spoon the beans over the toast and serve right away.

VARIATION

CHICKPEAS ON TOAST Omit the onion. Use chickpeas instead of navy beans, tahini for tomato paste, minced garlic for the syrup, lemon juice for cider vinegar, paprika for mustard, and cumin for soy sauce. No need to cook—though you certainly can; just stir everything to combine, mashing the chickpeas a bit with a fork, and serve on toast.

POSSIBLE TOPPINGS FOR TOAST OR HOT OR COLD CEREAL

- Fruit Compote (page 222)
- Plums, quartered and cooked over low heat until juicy
- Strawberries, roughly mashed and mixed with a squeeze of fresh lemon
- Cranberries, cooked with a little sugar until they burst
- Chopped orange or tangerine segments
- Red or Green Cooked Salsa (page 239)
- Pico de Gallo (page 236) or other fresh salsa
- Sautéed mushrooms
- Caramelized onions or shallots
- Leftover cooked greens

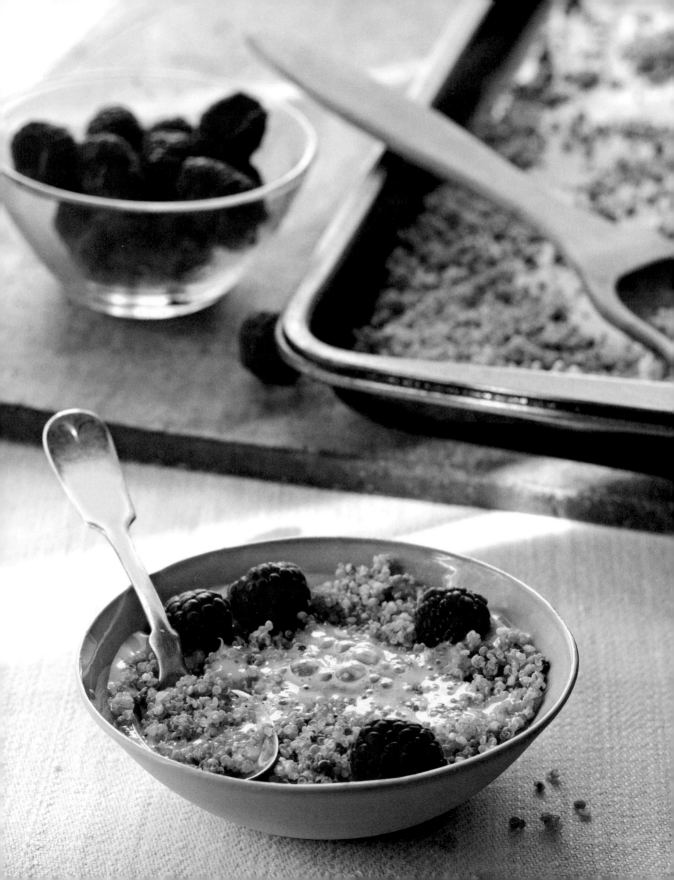

GRAIN NUTS WITH FRUIT

MAKES **4 servings**   TIME **About 20 minutes with precooked grains**

Twice-cooked grains translate to a one-ingredient breakfast cereal, along the lines of Grape-Nuts, but made by you and with zero extraneous ingredients. Name the grain and it can be served cereal fashion, which means you can use whatever you have leftover in the fridge, in whatever quantity (reduce the salt proportionately). The results: an intensely flavored breakfast cereal that is pleasantly dense and crunchy enough to sit in milk for a while without getting soggy.

2 cups cooked grain (any kind, like quinoa, bulgur, or wheat berries)

¼ teaspoon salt

4 cups diced fruit or berries

2 cups unsweetened plain non-dairy milk

1 Heat the oven to 375°F. Spread the grain on a large rimmed baking sheet, using your hands to break up any clumps and making the layer as even as possible. Sprinkle with the salt.

2 Bake, tossing once or twice with a spatula, until the grains dry out and turn golden brown, 15 to 25 minutes, depending on the size of the kernel and how crunchy you want them. Set the pan on a wire rack to cool.

3 Serve like breakfast cereal, with fruit either on top or in the bottom of the bowl and the milk poured over all.

MORE IDEAS

Instead of fruit, try topping with nuts or toasted coconut. • Add toasted sesame or pumpkin seeds.

DIY NON-DAIRY MILK

To make vegan milk at home: Put 1 cup of unsweetened shredded coconut or nuts in a blender with 2 cups boiling water; if using rolled oats or other rolled grains, increase the water to 6 cups and work in batches if you must. Pulse the machine on and off to help prevent the hot liquid from spurting out the top. Then hold the top on tightly and let the blender run for at least 15 seconds. Allow the mixture to steep for 15 minutes; then strain, preferably through cheesecloth, pressing on the solids to squeeze out as much milk as possible. Put the milk in a jar with a tight lid (discard the solids) and refrigerate for up to a week.

COCO-OAT-NUT GRANOLA

MAKES 18 ½-cup servings   TIME About 30 minutes

Increasingly, store-bought granolas are made from real ingredients—a good thing—but they still often include unnecessary sugars and calorie-dense dried fruits and often oil, which I've never found necessary. My simple five-ingredient granola is easy to prepare in large batches.

5 cups rolled oats (not quick-cooking or instant)

1 teaspoon ground cinnamon

½ teaspoon salt

1 cup unsweetened shredded coconut

3 cups chopped walnuts

1   Heat the oven to 350°F. Combine the oats and cinnamon in a large bowl; sprinkle with the salt. Toss well.

2   Spread the mixture on a rimmed baking sheet and bake for 30 minutes or a little longer, stirring occasionally so the granola browns evenly; adjust the temperature as necessary. The darker the oats get without burning, the crunchier the granola will be.

3   Remove the pan from the oven and add the coconut and walnuts. Put the pan on a wire rack to cool, stirring now and then, until the granola reaches room temperature. Serve with fresh fruit and an alternative milk or eat it out of hand. (Store in a sealed container in the fridge for a month or the freezer for several months.)

VARIATION

MUESLI   The no-bake version of granola. Combine the oats, walnuts, coconut, and cinnamon in a large bowl and sprinkle with salt. Toss well. Serve with fresh fruit or an alternative milk. (Store the muesli as you would granola.)

MORE IDEAS

Swap rolled wheat, rye, or kamut for the oats. • Skip the walnuts or substitute pecans, almonds, hazelnuts, or cashews. • Instead of the nuts, toss in sunflower, pumpkin, or sesame seeds. • Use ginger or cardamom instead of the cinnamon.

P.B. & J. COUSCOUS

MAKES 4 servings   TIME About 30 minutes

Couscous is actually a type of pasta that cooks and is eaten like a grain—
only it's even faster, lighter, and fluffier, which makes it the perfect vehicle
for this classic flavor combination. Seedless red grapes tend to be sweeter
than their tart green cousins, and seed-in grapes are the most flavorful,
so if you've got some time to kill to pit them, you'll be rewarded.

1⅓ cups whole wheat
couscous

½ teaspoon salt

3 cups seedless red grapes,
chopped

1 cup unsweetened plain
non-dairy milk (optional)

½ cup chopped unsalted
roasted peanuts

1   Put the couscous, salt, and 3 cups water in a medium pot over high
heat. Bring to a boil, stir in the grapes, then cover and remove from the
heat. Let stand, covered, for at least 10 minutes or up to 20 minutes.

2   Fluff the couscous with a fork. Serve topped with the milk if you like,
and the peanuts sprinkled on top.

MORE IDEAS

Add or swap nuts, like hazelnuts, walnuts, pistachios, pecans, pine nuts,
or coconut, for the peanuts. • Try different fruits, such as berries, mango,
peach, or banana.

WALK-AWAY OATMEAL

MAKES 4 servings   **TIME** 30 minutes

You can literally ignore this pot of oatmeal as it cooks, giving you more time to prepare for the day. This method is perfect for steel-cut oats— the unflattened version of rolled oats—which provide a chewier, denser cereal. As with any oatmeal porridge, you control how soupy or dry the results are by adding more or less water.

1½ cups steel-cut oats

½ teaspoon salt

1   Heat the oven to 350°F. Put the oats and salt in a medium ovenproof saucepan. If you want fluffy and dry oatmeal, add 2½ cups water; for thick porridge, use 3½ cups. Bring to a boil, stir, then cover the pot (with foil if you don't have a tight-fitting lid), and transfer to the oven.

2   Bake, undisturbed, for 20 minutes. Remove the oatmeal from the oven, stir, then cover it again and let it rest for another 5 minutes. Taste and add the desired seasonings or toppings from the ideas here or page 59 and serve immediately.

VARIATION

AUTUMN SPICE BAKED OATMEAL Like pumpkin pie for breakfast. Add 1 cup pureed pumpkin, 1 tablespoon maple syrup, 1 teaspoon cinnamon, and ¼ teaspoon nutmeg to the pot in Step 1. Top with chopped walnuts or pecans.

MORE IDEAS

Use quinoa or short-grain brown rice instead of oats. • Instead of water, cook the oats in unsweetened plain non-dairy milk. • Add maple syrup or other sweetener to the pot before—or after—baking. • Top with fresh or dried fruit. • Sprinkle with unsweetened shredded coconut and chopped mango. • Top with nuts before serving. • Serve with a drizzle of soy sauce and some sliced scallions. • Replace half of the water with salsa (see page 239).

SPICED BULGUR PILAF

MAKES 4 servings   **TIME** About 1 hour

Since it's already partially cooked, bulgur—which is steamed and dried cracked wheat—is super-fast to prepare. Medium is the most common grind and works well here, but if you find coarse bulgur, use that: The texture is very chewy and satisfying.

2 tablespoons pine nuts

2 tablespoons chopped almonds

2 tablespoons olive oil

1 cup bulgur

1 teaspoon ground cinnamon

¼ teaspoon ground nutmeg or allspice

¼ cup raisins or other chopped dried fruit

½ teaspoon salt

1 cup fresh orange juice

2 large apples (any kind), chopped

4 scallions, chopped (optional)

1 Set a large, deep skillet or medium saucepan over medium-high heat. Add the pine nuts and almonds and toast, shaking the pan frequently to avoid burning, until they're lightly browned and fragrant, 1 or 2 minutes. Remove the nuts from the pan.

2 Add the oil to the pan and when it's hot, add the bulgur, cinnamon, and nutmeg. Cook, stirring constantly until fragrant, less than 1 minute. Add the raisins, salt, orange juice, and 1 cup water and bring to a boil. Reduce the heat to a gentle bubble and cover the pan.

3 Cook, undisturbed, until most of the liquid is absorbed and the bulgur is just tender, 5 to 10 minutes. Uncover, stir in the apples and scallions if you like, and add a little more water if the grain is sticking to the bottom. Replace the lid, and remove from the heat. Let the pilaf rest for at least 5 minutes or up to 20 minutes. Taste, add the pine nuts and more salt if necessary, fluff with a fork, and serve hot or warm.

MORE IDEAS

Use whatever nuts you like. • Try strawberries, blueberries, peaches, plums, or pear instead of the apple. • Want it a bit spicier? Peel and mince a 2-inch piece of ginger and add it with the cinnamon in Step 2.

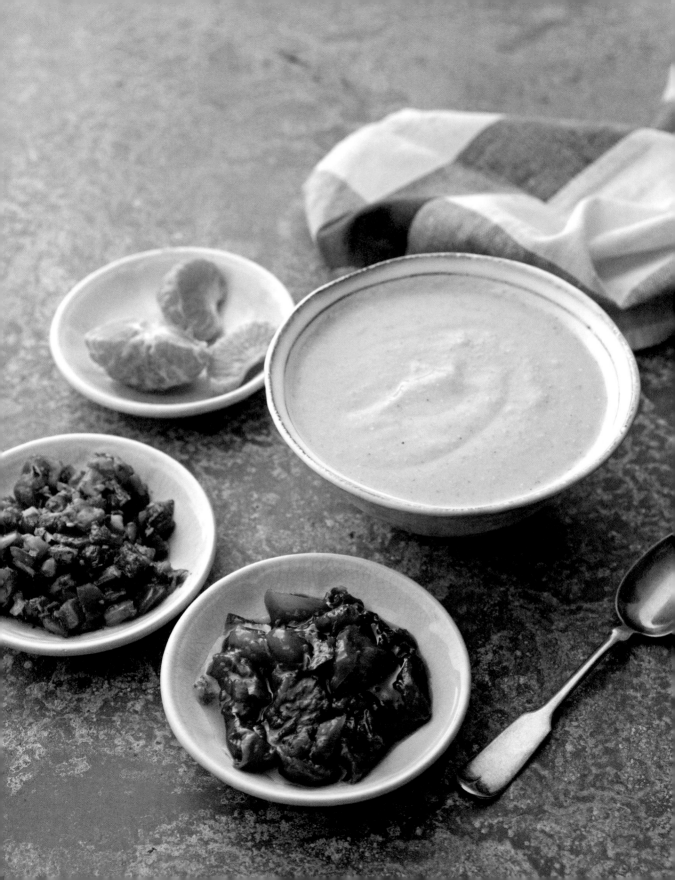

CORNMEAL MUSH WITH MANY TOPPINGS

MAKES 4 servings   **TIME** 30 to 40 minutes

The American name for polenta, cornmeal mush is a classic breakfast in this country. The coarser the cornmeal, the sturdier—and more textured—the results. (I like quite coarse cornmeal for this, though it does take an extra 5 to 10 minutes to cook.) See page 59 for topping ideas, both sweet and savory.

1 cup cornmeal, fine, medium, or coarse grind

½ cup unsweetened plain non-dairy milk

1 teaspoon salt

1   Put the cornmeal and 1 cup water in a medium pot and use a whisk to beat to a lump-free slurry. Whisk in the milk and the salt and set the pot over medium-high heat.

2   When the mixture starts to boil, lower the heat to medium and cook, whisking frequently and adding more water a little at a time to prevent lumps and keep the mixture loose, 15 to 30 minutes. Expect to add another 2½ to 3½ cups of water before the mush is ready. It will be thick and creamy, with just a little bite, and the mixture will pull away from the sides of the pan when you stir.

3   While the mush cooks, prepare your preferred topping. Serve hot in shallow bowls, with your choice of topping spooned over the surface.

VARIATION

FRIED CORNMEAL MUSH Cook the cornmeal a little longer than you would otherwise; it should be quite stiff. Transfer it to a greased standard-size (9 by 5-inch) loaf pan and refrigerate until cold and firm, at least 1 hour or up to a couple days. Invert the loaf onto a cutting board and cut into 8 slices. Heat 1 tablespoon olive oil in a nonstick skillet over medium heat. Fry 4 slices of the mush, turning once, until crisp and golden on both sides, 3 to 5 minutes. Repeat with the remaining pieces. Serve with any of the toppings on page 59.

MORE IDEAS

Oatmeal cooked like this is super-soft and creamy. So is cracked wheat (be sure not to confuse this with bulgur, which is precooked).

ALMOND QUINOA

MAKES 4 servings   **TIME** About 20 minutes

A rich, hot breakfast cereal, this is also delicious cold out of the fridge later in the week—it will taste like pudding. Eat it plain or, even better, top with fresh berries or juicy chopped fruit like pears or mango.

⅓ cup chopped almonds

2 cups unsweetened plain almond milk

1⅓ cups quinoa, rinsed and drained

½ teaspoon salt

2 tablespoons maple syrup (optional)

1 Put the almonds in a medium saucepan over medium-low heat and toast, shaking the pan occasionally, until they're fragrant, 3 to 5 minutes. Remove from the pot.

2 Put the milk, quinoa, and salt in the same pot along with ⅔ cup water and stir. Raise the heat to high and bring to a boil. Reduce the heat so the mixture bubbles steadily, cover, and cook undisturbed until most of the liquid is absorbed, 15 to 20 minutes.

3 Fluff the quinoa with a fork, turn off the heat, and let sit another 5 minutes. Sprinkle the almonds over the top, drizzle with syrup if you like, and serve right away or refrigerate for up to a week.

VARIATIONS

HAZELNUT QUINOA Swap hazelnut milk for almond milk and toasted hazelnuts for toasted almonds.

COCONUT QUINOA Substitute coconut milk for half the almond milk (reduced-fat is fine or use any other non-dairy milk here) and toasted unsweetened shredded coconut for the almonds.

MORE IDEAS

Try cracked wheat or steel-cut oats cooked this way.

BLUEBERRY SPOONBREAD

MAKES 4 servings   TIME 40 minutes

You often see breakfast tamales in Mexico, but few of us have the time
to mix, stuff, wrap, and steam tamales in the morning. Happily there's
a faster way to enjoy that same great mixture, only here with lots of
blueberries, too.

1 cup cornmeal

1½ cups hot water, or more
as needed

2 tablespoons olive oil

½ teaspoon salt

¼ teaspoon grated nutmeg

4 cups fresh or frozen
blueberries

Juice of 1 lemon

2 tablespoons maple syrup
(optional)

½ teaspoon baking powder

1 Heat the oven to 400°F. Combine the cornmeal, hot water, olive
oil, salt, and nutmeg; stir with a fork until smooth. Let it sit while you
prepare the blueberries.

2 Put the fruit, lemon juice, and syrup in a large ovenproof skillet
over medium-high heat. Cook, stirring occasionally, until the berries
start to release their juice, 5 to 10 minutes, depending on whether they
were frozen.

3 Stir the baking powder into the cornmeal mixture until it's completely incorporated. The mixture should be the consistency of thick
pancake batter; if it's too stiff, add a little more water. Spoon the batter
on top of the blueberries and spread it around with the back of a spoon;
it doesn't have to be perfect and it won't cover the whole top. Bake until
the topping has cracked and turned golden and is cooked all the way
through (a toothpick inserted into only the cornbread should come out
clean), 20 to 25 minutes. Spoon into shallow bowls and serve hot or at
room temperature.

MORE IDEAS

Try making the cornmeal batter with masa harina, the same stuff used to
make corn tortillas and authentic tamales. • Blackberries, boysenberries,
plums, apricots, peaches, mangos, or tomatoes (especially green tomatoes)
are all good options for the fruit. • Add fresh herbs to the batter. Try 1 teaspoon chopped thyme, rosemary, or basil. • Add up to ½ cup finely chopped
almonds, hazelnuts, or pistachios to the batter. • Go savory: Use chopped
fresh tomatoes, bell peppers, chiles, or scallions (or a combination) instead
of the blueberries. Omit the sugar and season with salt and pepper. • Go
sweeter: Drizzle the top with maple syrup before serving.

VB6 JOOK

MAKES 4 servings   TIME About 3 hours, largely unattended

This Chinese-style porridge—also known as congee or rice gruel—is made in many variations across Asia. I like using nontraditional brown rice with the classic toppings. A savory, extra-flavorful bowlful is a great alternative to oatmeal in the morning, and a double batch can last you and your family through the week. And with the variety of toppings and garnishes, you'll never feel like you're eating the same meal twice.

¾ cup short-grain brown rice

1 teaspoon salt

2 inches ginger, peeled

10 shiitake mushrooms, fresh or dried

4 teaspoons sesame oil

Soy sauce

1 cup chopped scallions, for garnish

½ cup fresh cilantro, for garnish

½ cup chopped roasted peanuts, for garnish

Rice vinegar or Chinese black vinegar, for garnish

1   Rinse the rice and put it in a large pot with 6 cups water and the salt. Bring to a boil over high heat, then turn the heat to low; the mixture should simmer, but only gently. Slice half the ginger and add it to the pot; mince the remaining ginger for adding later. If you're using fresh shiitakes, stem them (discard the stems or reserve for stock), slice the caps, and add them to the pot. If you're using dried shiitakes, cover them with boiling water and soak until pliable; discard the stems, then slice the caps and add to the pot.

2   Partially cover the pot and simmer for 2½ to 3 hours, stirring occasionally to make sure the rice is not sticking to the bottom. If it becomes very thick too quickly, turn down the heat and stir in more water. (You could need up to 2 cups more liquid in total.)

3   When the porridge is done, it will be soupy and creamy, like loose oatmeal. Add the minced ginger, the sesame oil, and soy sauce to taste. Serve with whichever garnishes you prefer.

VARIATIONS

SUPER VEGETABLE PORRIDGE When the porridge is thick but the rice is still a little underdone in Step 2, add 1 cup chopped napa cabbage or bok choy, ½ cup peas, and 1 chopped carrot. Return the lid and cook, stirring occasionally, until the vegetables are as tender as you like them, then proceed with Step 3.

PORRIDGE FOR DINNER Prepare the variation above or include some of the vegetables from the ideas below and add 1 cup diced chicken, beef, pork, or hard-boiled eggs along with the garnishes in Step 3.

MORE IDEAS

Top with diced tofu (smoked is especially nice). • Try other garnishes, alone or in combination, like bean sprouts, sliced celery, grated carrots, roasted garlic cloves, or thinly sliced raw button mushrooms. • Go sweet: Instead of the savory garnishes, use maple syrup, fresh (or a little dried) fruit, and nuts.

SCRAMBLED SWEET AND HOT PEPPERS

MAKES 4 servings　　**TIME** About 30 minutes

Every once in a while I want a blast of flavor in the morning—and this delivers, with a sweet heat that's completely addictive. Take it on the go, wrapped in a whole wheat flour tortilla, or eat it at home over whole-grain toast or a scoop of brown rice.

2 tablespoons olive oil

1 small onion, chopped

2 red bell peppers, chopped

1 large poblano chile, chopped

1 fresh hot chile (like jalapeño), chopped, or to taste

1 tablespoon minced garlic

1 teaspoon salt

½ teaspoon pepper

1½ pounds firm tofu (1½ blocks)

1　Put the oil in a large skillet over medium-high heat. Add the onion and cook, stirring occasionally, until it's translucent, 1 or 2 minutes.

2　Add the peppers, chiles, and garlic and sprinkle with the salt and pepper. Cook, stirring occasionally, until the peppers are brightly colored but not too soft, 3 to 5 minutes.

3　Crumble the tofu into the pan and stir, using a spatula to scrape the bottom of the pan and combine the tofu and vegetables; adjust the heat as necessary to avoid burning. When the mixture starts to stick to the pan, taste and adjust the seasoning and serve hot or warm.

BROCCOLI SCRAMBLE

MAKES 4 servings   **TIME** About 30 minutes

The one thing I sometimes miss in the morning is eggs, but tofu cooked like this comes pretty close, is equally quick, and is really satisfying—so much so that I crave it. Be sure to check out the variations below and the related recipe on page 71.

2 tablespoons olive oil

1 small red onion, halved and thinly sliced

1 pound broccoli, cut into florets

1 teaspoon salt

½ teaspoon pepper

1½ pounds firm tofu (1½ blocks), drained

1 tablespoon fresh lemon juice

1 Put the oil in a large skillet over medium-high heat. Add the onion and cook, stirring occasionally, until it's translucent, 1 or 2 minutes.

2 Add the broccoli and ¼ cup water and sprinkle with the salt and pepper. Cook, stirring occasionally, until the broccoli is brightly colored but still crisp and the pan is dry, 3 to 5 minutes.

3 Crumble the tofu into the pan and stir, using a spatula to scrape the bottom of the pan and combine the tofu and vegetables; adjust the heat as necessary to avoid burning. When the mixture starts to stick to the pan, add the lemon juice, taste and adjust the seasoning, and serve hot or warm.

VARIATION

TOMATO SCRAMBLE WITH SOY SAUCE Substitute 1 tablespoon sesame oil and 1 tablespoon vegetable oil for the olive oil, 1 bunch scallions for the red onion, and chopped tomatoes for the broccoli. In Step 2, cook the tomatoes until they release their liquid and the pan is dry, 5 to 10 minutes. Then proceed with the recipe; finish with soy sauce instead of lemon juice.

MORE IDEAS

This works for virtually any chopped or sliced vegetable—asparagus, peppers, mushrooms, spinach or other greens, cauliflower, you name it. Just adjust the cooking time in Step 2 accordingly. • For an added kick, throw in a pinch of cayenne, ground red chile, or fresh chile just before serving. • Try silken tofu for a completely different texture. (It comes in various degrees of firmness; see page 113 for an explanation.)

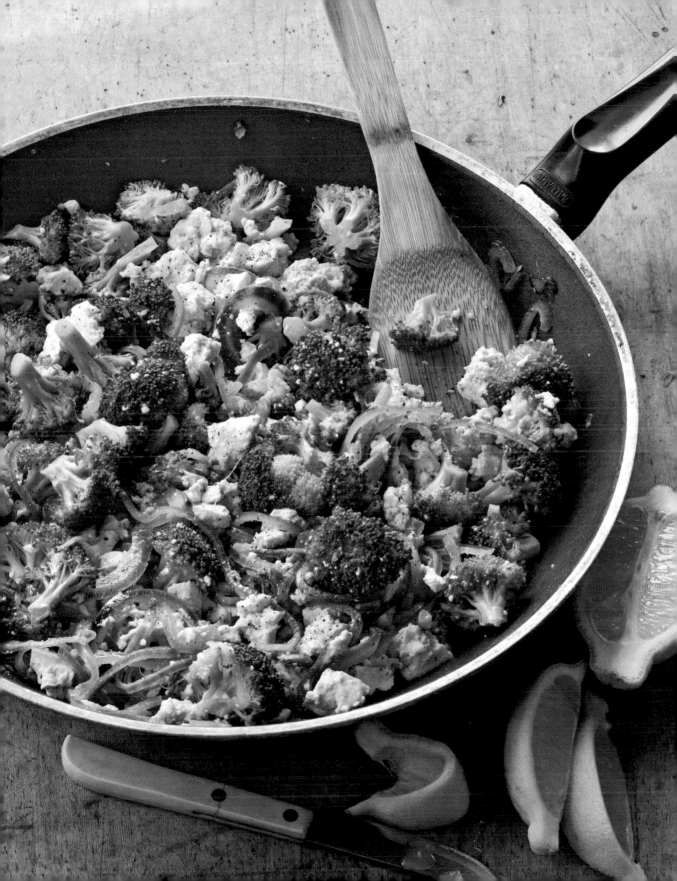

GOOD MORNING SWEET POTATO

MAKES 4 servings   **TIME** 20 minutes

So tell me why sweet potatoes haven't become popular for breakfast, really the most dessertlike meal of the day. The main recipe will remind you of Thanksgiving; for one savory and a less-sweet option, see the first two variations that follow. And if you don't have a microwave, the last variation has you covered.

4 sweet potatoes (about 2 pounds), scrubbed

1 cup chopped walnuts

¼ cup maple syrup or other sweetener

¼ teaspoon salt

1 Pierce each sweet potato in several places with a fork. Put them on a heatproof plate and cook in a microwave oven on high, stopping to turn them once or twice, until the centers are easily pierced with a small knife, 10 to 15 minutes.

2 Meanwhile, put the walnuts, syrup, salt, and ¼ cup water in a small saucepan over medium-low heat. Cook, stirring frequently, until the nuts are coated and fragrant.

3 When the potatoes are ready, slit the top of each lengthwise through the skin, just shy of both ends. Then squeeze the two ends between your fingers to mash some of the flesh and push it up through the opening. Nestle the nuts into the pulp on top and serve right away.

VARIATIONS

SALSA SWEET POTATO Skip the walnuts and syrup. Instead, warm 2 cups of any cooked salsa (see page 239 for a couple) to ladle into the potatoes.

SWEET CORN SWEET POTATO Instead of the nuts, put 2 cups fresh or frozen corn kernels and ¼ cup water into a small pot with the maple syrup in Step 2. Cook, stirring occasionally until caramelized, 3 to 5 minutes. Spoon into the potatoes.

ROASTED GOOD MORNING SWEET POTATO If you have the time, this is even better. Heat the oven to 425°F. Put the pierced sweet potatoes on a rimmed baking sheet and roast, turning once or twice, until their centers can be easily pierced with a small knife, 50 to 60 minutes.

MASTERING THE MICROWAVE

I'm not saying you should prepare whole meals in the microwave, but since a big part of living VB6 involves prepurposing—and reheating—leftovers and components you've made in advance, I'm hoping that singing the praises of these ubiquitous machines will inspire you to do more big-batch and make-ahead cooking, and incorporate more cooked vegetables—like this sweet potato—into your day. Here are three good reasons to use one.

You can eat a hot lunch: Almost every office has a microwave; all you need are microwave-safe containers and a commitment to eat a better midday meal. In the long run, you'll be saving yourself time and money—and chances are you'll feel better all afternoon.

Nor is this a life sentence of endless leftovers. You can quickly create inviting dishes on the fly by combining freshly cooked and cooked components (like vegetables, beans, or grains) with high-flavor ingredients (like herbs, spices, olive oil, or lemon juice). Invite co-workers to brown-bag it with you so you don't have to eat alone, or better still, organize conference room potlucks and working lunches.

Steaming is a breeze: It's a great way to cook vegetables, fish, chicken, and tofu (see page 113). You don't need special equipment, just a plate with a microwave-proof bowl inverted on top (or vice versa, if you prefer). You can be eating in the time it takes to heat the oven or boil a pot of water. Spend 30 minutes prepping and cooking vegetables at home, and you can stock the fridge with days' worth of food.

It's quick to eat from the freezer: Get into the habit of making extra and packing it into portion sizes you know you'll use; that way you'll ensure that you always have convenient meals for even the most hectic nights. Most microwave ovens have defrost settings, which might not work well for cuts of meat but are perfect for thawing and cooking frozen soups, stocks, stews, grains, beans—and, yes, leftovers.

GREEN APPLE STIR-FRY WITH CASHEWS

MAKES 4 servings   TIME 20 minutes

Some mornings demand a dish that blurs the line between sweet and savory, where the natural sweetness of fruit is enhanced with just a little salt. Enter this stir-fry, which comes together as quickly as a fruit salad and is equally good chilled or at room temperature, so it travels well to work and leftovers need never go to waste. You can chop the nuts and apples a bit if you'd prefer, but I find that large pieces are satisfying (and I eat them more slowly). Either way, serve it over toast, plain brown rice, or steel-cut oats—or nothing at all.

1 cup whole cashews

2 tablespoons olive oil

5 or 6 apples (about 1½ pounds), cut into wedges

½ teaspoon salt

1 tablespoon minced ginger

2 tablespoons fresh lemon juice

½ teaspoon pepper (optional)

1 Put the cashews in a large skillet over medium heat. Toast, shaking the pan occasionally, until the nuts are fragrant and golden, 5 to 10 minutes. Remove them from the pan and raise the heat to high.

2 Add the oil to the skillet. When it's hot, add the apples and salt, and cook undisturbed until the edges of the fruit begin to brown. Add the ginger to the pan and stir constantly with a spatula until the fruit begins to soften but hasn't begun to break up too much, 2 or 3 minutes.

3 Add the lemon juice and ¼ cup water. Stir and turn off the heat. Continue to stir occasionally, scraping up any browned bits from the bottom of the pan, until the liquid is almost absorbed. Add the cashews, and the pepper if you're using it, and stir. Taste and adjust the seasoning and serve.

VARIATIONS

PLUM STIR-FRY WITH PECANS Perfect for when plums aren't quite ripe yet. Pit the fruit and cut it into halves or wedges depending on how large they are. Use ½ teaspoon cardamom instead of the ginger and wait to add it until the plums are almost done.

APRICOT STIR-FRY WITH ALMONDS Take advantage of this natural affinity. Pit and halve the apricots. Skip the ginger and use ½ cup fresh orange juice instead of the lemon juice and water.

CANTALOUPE STIR-FRY WITH PISTACHIOS Or any melon, really. Seed and peel the melon and cut it into 1-inch chunks; figure 6 to 8 cups. Skip the ginger and swap lime juice for the lemon juice; and for something to wake up your taste buds, use a pinch of cayenne or other ground red chile instead of the black pepper.

GRAPEFRUIT STIR-FRY WITH COCONUT Sweet and sour in balance. Substitute unsweetened shredded coconut for the cashews; it will toast faster so watch it and keep the pan moving once it starts browning. Instead of the apples peel 4 grapefruits and divide them into segments, removing as many seeds as you can.

PINEAPPLE STIR-FRY WITH HAZELNUTS Chop the hazelnuts into large pieces. Peel and core a large pineapple and cut it into 1-inch chunks. Skip the ginger, but if you'd like add ¼ cup chopped fresh mint to the pineapple when you return the nuts to the skillet in Step 3.

MORE IDEAS

You get the idea from the variations. With the main recipe as your guide, almost any fruit and nut combination is possible.

SWEET RED BEAN BREAKFAST

MAKES 4 servings   TIME About 20 minutes

Take the best features of refried beans—the creaminess and the heft—and spin them in a breakfast direction. Then use them as you would a spreadable cheese, on apple wedges or whole-grain toast. Shockingly delicious.

3 cups cooked or canned pinto, kidney, or adzuki beans (see page 232)

¼ cup maple syrup

½ teaspoon ground cinnamon

½ teaspoon salt

4 green apples, sliced

1   Drain the beans. If you made them yourself, reserve the cooking liquid; if they're canned, discard it and rinse the beans.

2   Put the beans, syrup, cinnamon, salt, and ½ cup of the cooking liquid or water in a large saucepan over medium-high heat. Bring to a boil, then reduce the heat to a gentle bubble and cook, mashing with a fork or potato masher and adding just enough liquid to keep the mixture moist as you stir.

3   Continue to cook, stirring occasionally, until the beans thicken and begin to stick to the bottom of the pan, 4 to 6 minutes. Taste and adjust the seasoning and either eat with the apple slices once the beans cool off a bit or refrigerate for up to a week.

VARIATIONS

PEACHY BEAN BREAKFAST Swap white beans for red and use 1 chopped peach or pear in place of ¼ cup of the cooking liquid or water (to start; you may need to add more as the peaches cook). Reduce the syrup to 2 tablespoons (or skip it entirely).

CURRIED CHICKPEA BREAKFAST Use chickpeas instead of the red beans and substitute 2 teaspoons curry powder for the cinnamon.

MORE IDEAS

Use thick slices of jícama or radishes, or carrot or celery sticks, instead of (or in addition to) the apple slices.

NO-BAKE PUMPKIN CUSTARD

MAKES 4 servings   TIME 5 minutes, plus time for chilling if you like

The texture of this puddinglike breakfast is so creamy, you'll swear there's
dairy in here; and because it's not baked, it comes together in an instant.
For warm pumpkin custard, see the variations.

24 ounces silken tofu (about
3 cups)

One 15-ounce can pumpkin
puree

6 tablespoons maple syrup
or other sweetener

1 teaspoon vanilla extract

½ teaspoon ground
cinnamon

⅛ teaspoon salt

½ teaspoon ground ginger

¼ teaspoon ground nutmeg

1   Put all the ingredients in a food processor or a large bowl. Let the
machine run—or whisk by hand or with an electric mixer—until the tofu
is smooth and the pumpkin is fully incorporated.

2   Taste and adjust the seasoning. Serve right away or if you prefer,
chill the custard for a few hours (or overnight) in the fridge; it will
thicken a bit.

VARIATIONS

WARM, SWEET PUMPKIN SOUP Transfer the blended custard to
a saucepan over medium heat. When it just starts to bubble, begin
stirring constantly (this prevents splattering); cook until the mixture is
warmed all the way through, and serve.

FRESH PUMPKIN OR OTHER SQUASH CUSTARD This works for both
the chilled and warm versions. You can use your own puree from well-
drained roasted or steamed winter squash, like butternut, hubbard, or
acorn. Figure about 1½ cups.

MORE IDEAS

Pureed sweet potatoes, apples, plums, and pears all make good custards
with the same spices. • Top each serving with a sprinkling of chopped hazelnuts or pecans.

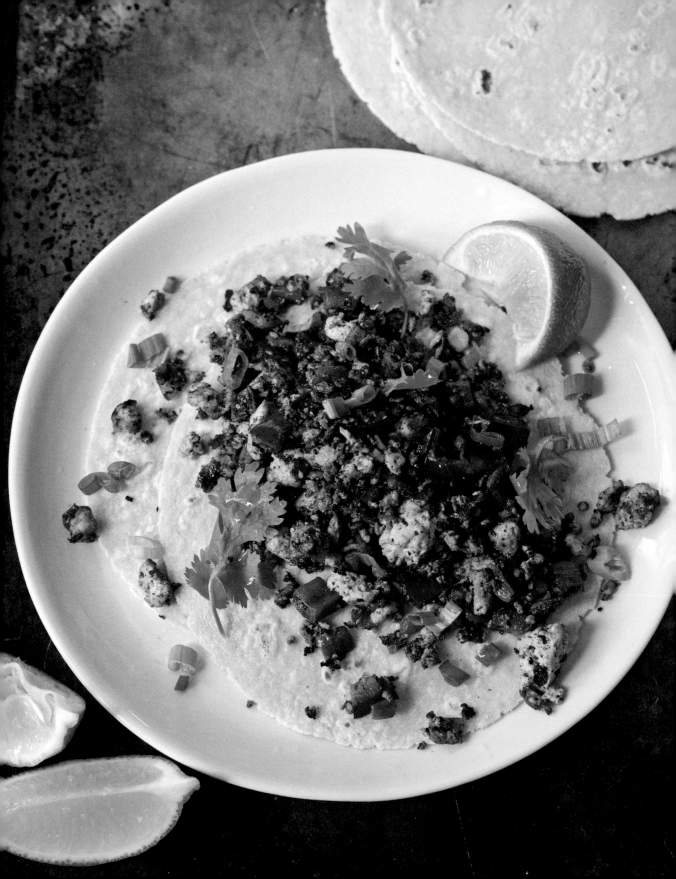

"CHORIZO" TACOS

MAKES 4 servings **TIME** 20 to 45 minutes, depending on the desired texture

Soft corn tortillas make a perfect vehicle for this tofu "chorizo," which is so good you'll find a lot of other uses for it too. Make it as soft or as crisp as you like, but use a nonstick pan for the best results; cast-iron is a good second choice. Since it's easy to double the batch well ahead of time, you might think about making this dish the next time you have a brunch.

Eight 6-inch corn tortillas

2 tablespoons olive oil

1 small red onion, chopped

1 tablespoon chopped garlic

1 teaspoon salt

½ teaspoon pepper

1½ pounds firm tofu
(1½ blocks)

1 red bell pepper, chopped
(optional)

1 tablespoon chili powder

2 limes, 1 halved,
1 quartered

¼ cup chopped fresh
cilantro, for garnish

¼ cup chopped scallions,
for garnish

1 Heat the oven to 400°F. Stack the tortillas on a large square of foil and wrap them loosely.

2 Put the oil in a large skillet over medium-high heat. Add the onion and garlic; sprinkle with the salt and pepper. Cook, stirring occasionally until the vegetables soften, 3 to 5 minutes.

3 Crumble the tofu into the pan with your hands. Cook, stirring and scraping the bottom of the skillet occasionally, and adjusting the heat as necessary, until the tofu browns and crisps as much or as little as you like it, anywhere from 10 to 30 minutes.

4 When the tofu is almost ready, put the tortillas in the oven.

5 Add the bell pepper to the pan if you're using it. Sprinkle the mixture with the chili powder; stir, and cook, continuing to scrape any browned bits from the bottom of the pan until the mixture is fragrant, less than a minute. Squeeze the juice of the halved lime over all, garnish with cilantro and scallions, and serve with the tortillas and lime quarters.

MORE IDEAS

For a little more kick without being too fiery, try 1 or 2 poblano chiles instead of the bell pepper. • Substitute 3 cups well-drained cooked or canned black or pinto beans for the tofu. (If you're using canned beans, rinse them before draining.) • Use tempeh instead of tofu. It will be tangier and slightly more dense, closer to the texture of ground meat. • Small whole wheat tortillas are good, here, too. Soften them the same way as described above.

CRISP QUINOA-CORN CAKES

MAKES 4 servings   TIME About 1 hour

Kitchen mistakes often become epiphanies: The first time I overcooked a batch of quinoa, I was disheartened. Now I use the fluffy, starchy, slightly sticky grains to help bind all sorts of egg-free cakes. (For another example, check out the Walnut Banana Bread on page 86.) In summer, make these with raw corn kernels cut straight from the cob. And leftovers—cold or warmed—make a terrific lunch on top of a big salad.

2 tablespoons olive oil

1 cup quinoa, rinsed and drained

1 teaspoon salt

½ teaspoon pepper

1 cup corn kernels (frozen are fine; don't bother to thaw)

½ cup chopped scallions or red onion

¼ cup chopped fresh cilantro

1 teaspoon cumin seeds

1 cup any fresh or cooked salsa (see pages 236 and 239 for some recipes)

1   Heat the oven to 425°F. Grease a baking sheet with 1 tablespoon of the oil. Put the quinoa in a large pot along with the salt. Add enough water to cover by about 1½ inches. Bring to a boil, then adjust the heat so the mixture bubbles gently.

2   Cook, stirring occasionally, until the quinoa is overcooked: The kernels should be so tender they burst and become starchy and are thick like mashed potatoes, 25 to 35 minutes. As they cook, adjust the heat and add small amounts of water to keep the bottom from burning without making the mixture soupy. When the quinoa is ready, cover, remove from the heat, and let it sit for 5 minutes.

3   Stir in the pepper, corn, scallions, cilantro, and cumin with a rubber spatula, mashing a bit to make the grains even stickier. When the mixture is cool enough to handle, scoop up about ¾ cup with your hands, form a 1-inch-thick cake, and transfer to the prepared pan. Repeat to make eight cakes.

4   Brush or smear the remaining 1 tablespoon of oil on top of the cakes and bake, turning once, until golden and crisp on both sides and hot in the center, 15 to 20 minutes. Let them cool in the pan a bit to set up, then serve warm with the salsa.

VARIATIONS

CRISP RICE AND PEA CAKES Super with a salad for dinner, especially if you add a little grated Parmesan to the cakes. Use short-grain brown rice instead of the quinoa, peas instead of the corn, and 1 tablespoon chopped garlic instead of the scallions. The rice will take 5 or 10 minutes longer than the quinoa to become overcooked and starchy.

MORE IDEAS

You can almost cook any grain this way: brown rice, bulgur, steel-cut oats, millet, even whole wheat couscous.

COCONUT HOECAKES WITH MANGO SALSA

MAKES **4 servings**   TIME **30 minutes**

Imagine eating warm, soft coconut macaroons topped with the creamiest, sweetest fruit on the planet and you have some idea of how good these hoecakes are.

2 large mangos, chopped

Juice of 1 lemon

½ cup unsweetened shredded coconut

1½ cups cornmeal

¼ teaspoon salt

1½ cups boiling water

3 tablespoons vegetable oil

1 Heat the oven to 350°F. Combine the mangos and lemon juice in a bowl and let it sit.

2 Spread the coconut on a rimmed baking sheet and cook, checking and stirring occasionally until fragrant and golden, 4 to 7 minutes. Remove to a bowl to cool. Turn the oven down to 200°F and put the empty baking sheet inside.

3 Combine the cornmeal and salt in a medium bowl. Gradually pour in the boiling water, whisking constantly. Let the mixture sit until the cornmeal absorbs the water, 5 to 10 minutes. Then stir in the coconut.

4 Coat a large skillet or griddle (nonstick or cast-iron, if you have it) with 1 tablespoon of the oil and put it over medium heat. When it's hot, add spoonfuls of the batter to the skillet or griddle, making any size cakes you like. (Be careful; it spatters a bit.) Cook until bubbles appear and burst on the top and the underside browns, 2 or 3 minutes; turn and cook on the other side until golden, another 2 or 3 minutes. Transfer the cakes to the pan in the warm oven and continue making hoecakes, adding some more of the remaining 2 tablespoons oil with each batch. Serve hot, topped with the mango mixture.

MORE IDEAS

Other fruits—strawberries, pineapple, bananas, peaches, pears, for example—all work well instead of the mangos. • To make these richer, use scalding hot unsweetened plain non-dairy milk instead of the boiling water. (You can use coconut milk for an even more intense flavor, but cut it by at least half with a grain or nut non-dairy milk.) • You can boost the sweet-and-salty profile here by adding chopped fresh cilantro or basil to the topping. A pinch of cayenne or other ground red chile will make it even more like fresh salsa.

BLUEBERRY OATMEAL PANCAKES

MAKES 4 servings   **TIME** 30 minutes with precooked oatmeal

These pancakes are an easy way to use up leftover oatmeal, but they're so good they're worth cooking up a fresh batch. If you don't have a cast-iron or nonstick skillet, be prepared to use more oil.

½ cup whole wheat flour

¼ cup rolled oats (not quick-cooking or instant)

1 teaspoon baking powder

½ teaspoon ground cinnamon

½ teaspoon salt

¾ cup unsweetened plain non-dairy milk, plus more if needed

1 teaspoon grated lemon zest

2 cups cooked oatmeal (made from rolled oats)

3 tablespoons vegetable oil

1½ cups blueberries (frozen are fine; thaw them first)

¼ cup maple syrup

1 Heat the oven to 200°F. Combine the flour, oats, baking powder, cinnamon, and salt in a large bowl.

2 In a smaller bowl, whisk together the milk and zest; stir in the cooked oatmeal until it's completely incorporated.

3 Add the oatmeal mixture to the flour mixture and stir gently; don't overmix. The mixture should be the consistency of thick pancake batter; if not, add either a little more milk or whole wheat flour as needed.

4 Put a large skillet or griddle over medium heat. When a few drops of water dance on its surface, add 1 tablespoon of the vegetable oil and let it get hot. Working in batches, spoon the batter onto the skillet or griddle, making any size pancakes you like; spread the batter around a bit so they're not too thick. Scatter some of the blueberries over the top of each; press them in gently. Cook until bubbles form on the top and pop, 3 to 4 minutes; you may have to rotate the cakes in the pan to cook them evenly, depending on your heat source and pan.

5 Carefully flip the pancakes and cook until they're browned on the other side, a couple of minutes more. As they finish, transfer them to a platter in the oven while you cook the remaining batter (adding more oil as necessary). Serve drizzled with maple syrup.

MORE IDEAS

Thinly sliced bananas, apples, or strawberries all are delicious options here, as are blackberries or raspberries.

APPLE-OAT MUFFINS

MAKES **12 servings**   TIME **About 45 minutes**

Fruit is the key to healthy vegan baking. It adds moisture, body, and sweetness—things for which you would otherwise rely on eggs, butter, and sugar. You don't have to use pastry flour if you don't have it handy, but it does make the crumb a little lighter and fluffier.

½ cup vegetable oil

5 or 6 apples (about 1½ pounds, any type but red delicious)

½ cup maple syrup or other sweetener

⅓ cup (3½ ounces) silken tofu

½ cup unsweetened plain non-dairy milk

1½ cups whole wheat flour, preferably pastry flour

1 cup rolled oats (not quick-cooking or instant)

2 teaspoons baking powder

½ teaspoon ground cardamom

¼ teaspoon baking soda

¼ teaspoon salt

1 Heat the oven to 375°F and grease two 6-cup muffin tins with some of the oil or fill with liners. Peel the apples and shred them on a box grater, turning them as you work; discard the cores. Put the shredded apple in a strainer and press down to extract as much liquid as possible. You should have about 1½ cups packed grated apples.

2 Put the syrup, tofu, and milk in a small bowl and whisk until smooth and foamy. Combine the flour, oats, baking powder, cardamom, baking soda, and salt in a large bowl. Fold the wet mixture into the dry mixture, add the apples, and stir until just combined; don't overdo it or the muffins will be tough.

3 Divide the batter among the prepared cups or liners, pressing down gently to fill them completely. It's okay if they're mounded a little. Bake until the muffins are puffed, golden brown on top, and springy to the touch, 30 to 35 minutes. Serve warm if possible (freeze the leftovers to reheat later).

WALNUT BANANA BREAD

MAKES **12 servings**   TIME **About 1 hour**

Whenever you have leftover brown rice and overripe bananas around, try this whole-grain banana bread packed with fruit, spices, and nuts. It's a real treat. As the loaf bakes, it forms a rice-flecked crust for a pleasant crunch and a contrast of textures in every bite. Serve it with some fresh berry jam (see page 58).

¼ cup vegetable oil

4 overripe large bananas

1½ cups cooked long-grain brown rice

¾ cup maple syrup

1 teaspoon vanilla extract

1½ cups whole wheat flour

2 teaspoons baking powder

½ teaspoon salt

1 teaspoon ground cinnamon

¼ teaspoon ground allspice

¼ teaspoon grated nutmeg

½ cup chopped walnuts

1   Heat the oven to 375°F. Grease a 9 by 5-inch loaf pan with some of the oil. Mash the bananas in a large bowl. Add the rice, maple syrup, vanilla, and the remaining oil; stir until thoroughly combined.

2   Put the flour, baking powder, salt, and spices in a medium bowl; stir until everything is evenly distributed.

3   Fold the dry ingredients into the rice mixture along with the nuts. Gently stir until the mixture is just combined.

4   Pour the batter into the prepared pan and bake for 45 to 50 minutes, or until a toothpick poked into the middle comes out clean. Let sit on a wire rack for 10 to 15 minutes before inverting, then cool completely before slicing. (Store loosely wrapped in the refrigerator for up to a day or two, or freeze in an airtight container for up to a couple months.)

VARIATIONS

SWEET POTATO-HAZELNUT BREAD Swap 3 small sweet potatoes—steamed, peeled, and mashed—for the bananas (you should have about 2 cups). Use hazelnuts instead of the walnuts.

DOUBLE-PUMPKIN BREAD Use 2 cups cooked or canned pumpkin and green pumpkin seeds instead of the bananas and nuts.

MORE IDEAS

Toss in dried raisins or cranberries along with the nuts. • Try other leftover cooked whole grains (like quinoa, oatmeal, or millet) instead of the rice. • Cooked and mashed apples, pears, or apricots work well in this bread too.

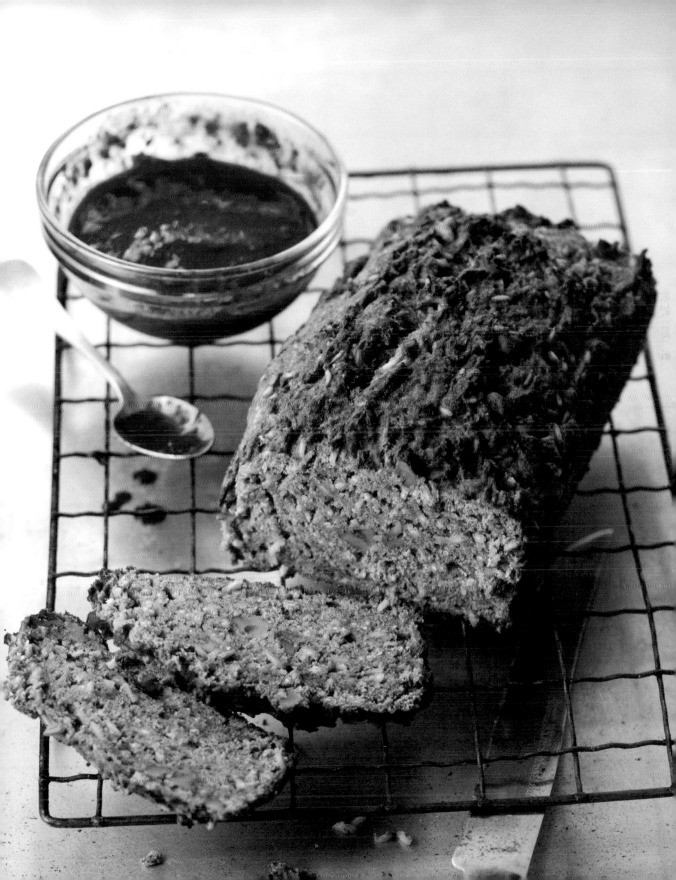

LUNCH

SWEETGREEN QUINOA SALAD

PEANUTTY CHOPPED SALAD

FAVA BEAN SALAD

TOFU CEVICHE

CHICKPEA TABBOULEH

PEAS AND CARROTS SALAD

MOROCCAN POTATO SALAD

RIBOLLITA

HEARTY MISO SOUP

CURRIED CARROT AND
LENTIL SOUP

RHUBARB AND RED LENTIL SOUP

ORANGE SOUP WITH BLACK
SALSA

CREAMY TOMATO SOUP

RED SOUP

GRAINS MARINARA

SPAGHETTI WITH BEAN
BOLOGNESE

SEAWEED SOBA

TOFU STEAKS WITH COLD
NOODLES

CAPONATA MIXED RICE

EDAMAME FRIED RICE

FULLY LOADED BEAN BURRITOS

CAULIFLOWER ROMESCO

CURRIED SPINACH AND TOFU

SLOW-COOKED BRUSSELS
SPROUTS WITH LEMONGRASS

TERIYAKI TEMPEH WITH
BOK CHOY

VEGETABLE POT PIE

EGGPLANT MEATBALLS

P.L.T. SANDWICH

PHONY BOLOGNA

MUSHROOM-NUT BURGERS
OVER GREENS

Any way you can cook or serve meat works just as well with vegetables—sometimes better, in fact.

Keep reminding yourself of this, especially at lunchtime, when you're wondering what to have instead of a cheeseburger. Whether you like to eat soup, a sandwich, salad, or pizza, there are lots of choices here, with all the variations and ideas you need to make your midday meal appealing.

I promise: Nothing in this chapter is difficult to make; and if you prepare only one meal a day, let this be it. Many of the dishes in this chapter are served in bowls: hearty soups, loaded salads, stir-fries to eat with or without rice or noodles. This is, after all, how much of the world eats, and it's a handy way to assemble meals that travel well. (For more on that, see the sidebar on page 75.) You'll also find a template for building a well-filled burrito and a simple vegan bologna (really!) that's head and shoulders above the hyper-processed sandwich fillings you'll find in the deli aisle. If you have a little more time, try the pot pie or meatballs. Almost everything in this chapter can be made ahead and reheated whenever and wherever you're ready to eat.

I always get asked about protein, so let me reassure you: Beans, grains, and even vegetables supply all you need. Period. And since I started eating vegan lunches, I find I have more energy in the afternoons and never get that bogged-down feeling that comes after a big meat-or-cheese and white-flour-heavy meal. If you're still concerned, focus on the tofu and tempeh recipes (and on the core tofu preparations on pages 240–41). You might become a convert.

Once you focus on the possibilities and the benefits instead of the limitations, I'm confident you'll see that switching to a plant-based lunch is not only no big deal, it's a pleasure.

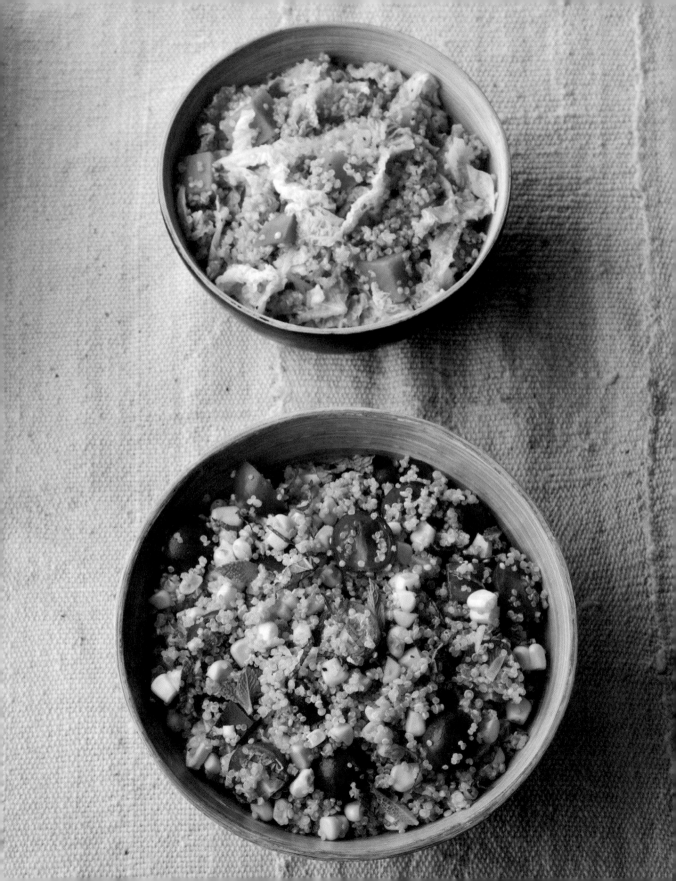

SWEETGREEN QUINOA SALAD

MAKES **4 servings**   TIME **20 minutes with cooked grains**

Long called a super-grain (it's actually not a grain but a chenopod, but let's not let that bother us), quinoa has become super-hip—to the point where supply is having a hard time keeping up with demand. You'll find it easily enough, though, and a little goes a long way, especially in a vegetable-driven salad like this. The main recipe is best in summer, when tomatoes and corn are at their peak. For rest-of-the-year options—including the springtime salad served in Sweetgreen restaurants to celebrate the publication of this book—see the ideas that follow.

2 tablespoons olive oil

2 tablespoons sherry or red wine vinegar

1 tablespoon Dijon mustard, or to taste

½ teaspoon salt

¼ teaspoon pepper

1 large shallot or small red onion, chopped

1 teaspoon minced garlic

3 cups cooked quinoa (see page 230)

1 large red bell pepper, chopped

2 cups corn kernels, preferably fresh

1 pint cherry or grape tomatoes, halved

1 cup chopped fresh basil or mint

1 Whisk together the oil, vinegar, mustard, salt, and pepper with 2 tablespoons water in a large bowl. Add the shallot and garlic, whisk again, and taste. Add more mustard if you like.

2 Add the remaining ingredients to the bowl and toss with a fork and spoon until everything is evenly coated in dressing. Taste and adjust the seasoning and serve right away, or refrigerate for up to an hour or so.

VARIATION

SWEETGREEN SEASONAL QUINOA SALAD Vary the vegetables according to what looks best in season. Greens or cabbage are always good choices. In winter, try tossing in leftover cooked vegetables straight from the fridge. Sweetgreen's spring version includes farro, asparagus, kale, arugula, tofu, toasted almonds, and other locally sourced vegetables. The fast vinaigrette in the main recipe here goes with virtually everything, but when you're in the restaurant, you can choose from several vegan dressings.

MORE IDEAS

A bold salad like this would also be great with any number of other grains: bulgur, millet, wheat berries, or farro, for example. Add crunch by tossing in toasted pine nuts, shelled pumpkin seeds, or sliced almonds. • Up the protein by adding black beans, chickpeas, or tofu. (For some crisp tofu ideas see the recipe and variations on pages 240–41.) • Year-round, use fresh parsley instead of basil, or skip the fresh herb entirely.

PEANUTTY CHOPPED SALAD

MAKES **4 servings**   TIME **30 minutes**

Chopped salad is a staple, and you can use literally any vegetable that you can eat raw. Taking the extra time to chop the greens and vegetables is always worth it, because dressing and ingredients become evenly distributed, and everything is much easier to eat. I almost never make salad any other way.

¼ cup peanut butter

2 tablespoons rice vinegar

1 teaspoon salt

½ teaspoon pepper

1 head romaine lettuce, chopped into bite-size pieces

2 carrots, chopped

4 celery stalks, chopped

1 small red onion, chopped

1 cucumber, peeled, seeded, and chopped

1 red bell pepper, chopped

8 to 10 radishes, chopped

1 Put the peanut butter, vinegar, salt, and pepper in a large bowl with ½ cup water; whisk until smooth.

2 Add the remaining ingredients, toss to coat in the dressing, and serve right away.

VARIATIONS

CHOPPED SALAD WITH TAHINI DRESSING Especially good mounded on top of thick tomato slices. Instead of the peanut butter use tahini, and substitute lemon juice for the rice vinegar.

DOUBLE-CRUNCHY COLE SLAW Swap almond butter for the peanut butter. Substitute 1 small head green cabbage for the lettuce, and omit the bell pepper and cucumber.

MORE IDEAS

Make the salad heartier by tossing in 1 cup cooked whole grains, like quinoa or wheat berries. • Add chopped fresh cilantro or mint before tossing. • For dinner, top with slices of grilled chicken, steak, pork loin, shrimp, or fish.

FAVA BEAN SALAD

MAKES 4 servings   **TIME** 10 minutes

We don't eat fava beans nearly as much as does the rest of the world—a shame, considering both the green immature and the big brown forms are so versatile. Maybe it's because fresh favas are a pain to shuck and peel. But you can avoid all that by using frozen or canned, or by cooking dried favas from scratch, as I do for this salad (see page 232).

3 cups cooked or canned mature fava beans (see page 232)

1 cucumber, peeled and seeded if you like, chopped

3 celery stalks, sliced

1 large shallot or small red onion, chopped

3 tablespoons olive oil

1 tablespoon fresh lemon juice, or more to taste

½ teaspoon salt

¼ teaspoon pepper

2 tomatoes, chopped

½ cup chopped fresh mint

¼ cup chopped fresh dill

1 Drain the beans; if they're canned, rinse them as well. Combine the beans with all the ingredients except the tomatoes and herbs in a large bowl. Stir and let sit for up to 1 hour or refrigerate for up to 1 day.

2 Just before serving stir in the tomatoes, mint, and dill, then taste and adjust the seasoning.

MORE IDEAS

Use frozen (or fresh shelled and skinned) green fava beans. Defrost them in the microwave or in a small pot of boiling water and quickly blanch before tossing with other ingredients. • Use other large beans instead of favas, like gigantes or flageolets. • Try thinly sliced fennel or raw artichoke instead of the celery (figure about 2 cups). • Swap orange segments for the tomatoes. • Use basil or parsley instead of the mint.

TOFU CEVICHE

MAKES **4 servings** TIME **20 minutes, plus pickling time**

Tofu is made a lot like cheese, so it doesn't require cooking. It does, however, benefit from marinating, and—within limits—the longer the better. There are so many ways to eat this refreshing dish: over greens, brown rice, or grains; with Boston lettuce leaves for wrapping; tossed with whole wheat angel hair; tucked into warm corn tortillas; or, of course, all on its own.

1½ pounds firm tofu (1½ blocks)

½ cup cider vinegar or sherry vinegar

1 teaspoon sugar

1 teaspoons salt

4 scallions, sliced

1 teaspoon minced garlic

1 bunch radishes, sliced or chopped

1 cucumber, sliced or chopped

1 avocado, cubed

1 tablespoon olive oil

½ teaspoon pepper

½ cup chopped fresh cilantro

1 Cut the tofu into small cubes. Put the vinegar, sugar, salt, and 1 cup water in a large bowl. Whisk to combine, then add the scallions, garlic, and tofu; toss gently to coat with the marinade. Refrigerate for as little as 15 minutes or up to 2 days.

2 Drain the tofu mixture, reserving the pickling liquid. Put the tofu mixture in a large bowl and add the radishes, cucumber, and avocado.

3 Toss the ceviche with 2 tablespoons of the reserved liquid, and the olive oil and pepper. Taste and adjust the seasoning, adding more pickling liquid if you like. Sprinkle with the cilantro and serve.

VARIATIONS

GREEK-STYLE TOFU CEVICHE Use red wine vinegar instead of cider. Swap 1 small red onion for the scallions, 2 tomatoes for the radishes, capers or chopped olives for the avocado, and parsley for the cilantro.

VIETNAMESE-STYLE TOFU CEVICHE Use lime juice instead of the vinegar and add 1 or 2 teaspoons fish sauce (unless you're being strictly vegan). Try fresh mint or Thai basil instead of the cilantro. Top with crushed peanuts if desired.

MORE IDEAS

Make it even more herbaceous by tossing in fresh basil and mint along with the cilantro.

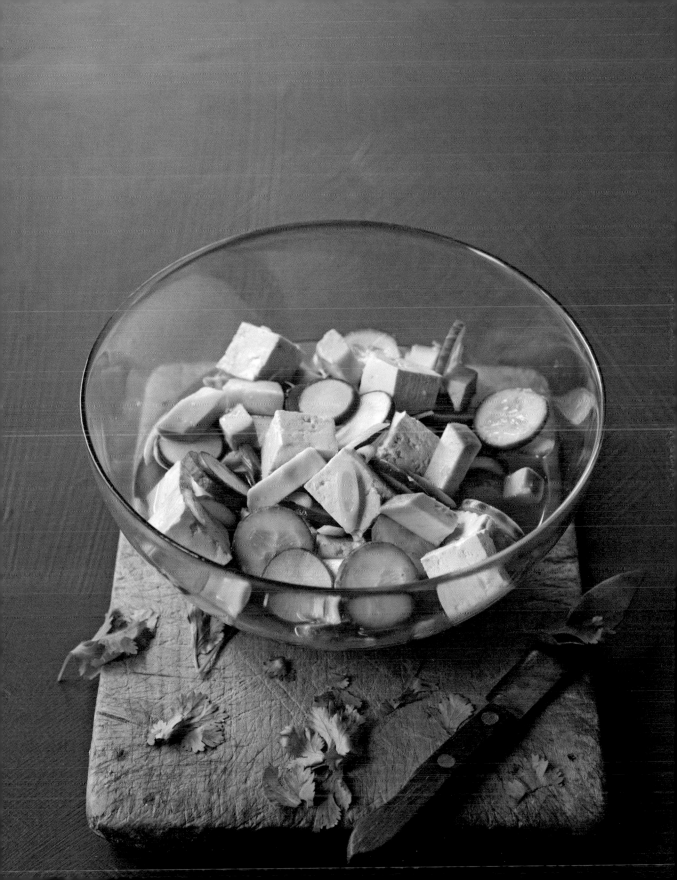

CHICKPEA TABBOULEH

MAKES 4 servings **TIME** 15 minutes

All tabbouleh is easy to make, but this version is even easier than most, and the texture of the mashed beans is similar to the bulgur used in the classic recipe. Feel free to improvise with any additional or alternative vegetables, including cooked leftovers. A few ideas: asparagus, peas, spinach, or eggplant, especially grilled.

3 cups cooked or canned chickpeas (see page 232)

2 large tomatoes, chopped

2 celery stalks (the leaves are good too), chopped

1 bell pepper, chopped

6 or 7 radishes, chopped

1 cup chopped fresh parsley

1 cup chopped fresh mint

½ cup chopped scallions

16 black olives, pitted and chopped (optional)

3 tablespoons olive oil

1 tablespoon fresh lemon juice, or more to taste

¼ teaspoon pepper

½ teaspoon salt

1 Drain the chickpeas; if they're canned, rinse them before draining. Put the chickpeas in a large bowl and mash with a fork or a potato masher until the beans break up a bit.

2 Add the remaining ingredients and toss until everything is combined and coated in dressing. Taste and adjust the seasoning, adding lemon juice as needed. Serve right away or refrigerate for up to 2 hours.

MORE IDEAS

Vary the legume. Try this with white beans, lentils, or thawed frozen beans like limas or black-eyed peas. • Substitute chopped pistachios or almonds, or toasted pine nuts, for some or all of the chickpeas. • Use chopped fresh basil or dill for some or all of the mint.

PEAS AND CARROTS SALAD

MAKES 4 servings   **TIME** 90 minutes, largely unattended

Add some substance to this classic combination and you have lunch. Hulled barley, also called barley groats, are the whole-grain form of barley, with the outer husk and bran layers intact. (Common pearled barley is more highly processed.) This form takes a little longer to cook, but just plan a bit ahead; it's worth it.

1 cup hulled barley

1½ teaspoons salt

3 tablespoons olive oil

1 large carrot, chopped

1 celery stalk, chopped

1 small onion, chopped

1 teaspoon chopped garlic

¼ teaspoon pepper

1½ cups fresh or frozen peas

1 tablespoon fresh lemon juice, or more to taste

¼ cup chopped fresh mint or parsley, for garnish

1 Rinse the barley and put it in a medium saucepan with water to cover by at least 2 inches. Add 1 teaspoon salt and bring to a boil. Lower the heat so the water bubbles gently, cover, and cook, stirring once in a while, until the barley is tender but not mushy, anywhere from 45 to 60 minutes.

2 Meanwhile, put 1 tablespoon of the oil in a large skillet over medium heat. When the oil is hot, add the carrot, celery, onion, and garlic; sprinkle with the remaining ½ teaspoon salt and the pepper and cook, stirring occasionally, until the vegetables just begin to soften, 3 to 5 minutes. Add the peas and stir until they're warmed, 1 or 2 minutes. Transfer the vegetables to a large bowl.

3 When the barley is ready drain it, shaking the strainer and fluffing it with a fork until it cools and dries a bit. Add the barley to the bowl with the vegetables along with the remaining 2 tablespoons olive oil and the lemon juice. Toss to combine, taste, and adjust the seasoning, adding more lemon juice if you'd like; garnish with the herbs and serve.

MORE IDEAS

Add some crunch by tossing in toasted pine nuts or almonds. • Make this salad creamy by using 2 tablespoons Vegannaise (page 242) or silken tofu instead of the olive oil In Step 3. • Add 1 pound firm tofu cubes in Step 2, with the peas.

MOROCCAN POTATO SALAD

MAKES 4 servings   TIME About 40 minutes

There are more vegetables in this salad than potatoes, which is not only how I've always preferred potato salad but, really, also a better way. The toasted spices, chickpeas, and raisins make this recipe exotic but not at all difficult to prepare. Serve it on a bed of fresh spinach for some bite and heft.

½ pound starchy potatoes (like russet), peeled and cut into ½-inch cubes

2 cups cooked or canned chickpeas

3 tablespoons olive oil

1 large onion, chopped

2 large carrots, chopped

1 tablespoon minced ginger

2 red bell peppers, chopped

¼ cup raisins

2 teaspoons cumin seeds

½ teaspoon ground cinnamon

¼ teaspoon pepper

1½ teaspoons salt

¼ teaspoon cayenne (optional)

2 tablespoons fresh lemon juice

Chopped fresh parsley, for garnish

1   Put the potatoes in a pot with enough water to cover by about 1 inch and bring to a boil. Cook, stirring once or twice, until fully tender and easily pierced with a fork, 10 to 15 minutes. Drain the potatoes and transfer to a large bowl.

2   Drain the chickpeas; if they're canned, rinse them before draining. Put 2 tablespoons of the olive oil in a large skillet over medium-high heat. When it's hot, add the onion, carrots, and ginger. Cook, stirring occasionally, until the vegetables begin to get tender, 3 to 5 minutes. Add the chickpeas along with the bell peppers, raisins, cumin, cinnamon, pepper, salt, and cayenne if you're using it. Stir until fragrant, 2 or 3 minutes, and remove from the heat.

3   Add the vegetables and spices to the potatoes along with the lemon juice, parsley, and the remaining 1 tablespoon olive oil. Stir until everything is combined and the potatoes break up a bit. Taste, adjust the seasoning, and serve warm or cold.

MORE IDEAS

Substitute chopped dried apricots for the raisins. • Add a salty element by tossing in ½ cup chopped pitted black or green olives or 1 tablespoon minced preserved lemon. • Make it spicier by replacing the cayenne with harissa—the not-too-hot seasoned chile paste from Morocco; you can find it in some supermarkets and most international groceries. Stir in 1 tablespoon (more or less to taste) in Step 2 instead of the cayenne.

RIBOLLITA

MAKES 4 servings   TIME About 40 minutes

Super-satisfying and completely traditional, this is a hearty Tuscan vegetable and bean stew served over a giant crouton. It's one of my favorite soups, period.

3 tablespoons olive oil

1 small onion, chopped

1 carrot, chopped

1 celery stalk, chopped

1 tablespoon minced garlic

1 teaspoon salt

½ teaspoon pepper

2 cups cooked or canned cannellini beans (see page 232)

One 15-ounce can whole peeled tomatoes

4 cups vegetable stock (see page 246) or water

1 fresh rosemary sprig

1 fresh thyme sprig

4 slices whole-grain bread, toasted

1 pound kale or escarole, chopped

1   Put the oil in a large pot over medium heat. When it's hot, add the onion, carrot, celery, and garlic, sprinkle with the salt and pepper and cook, stirring occasionally, until the vegetables are soft, 5 to 10 minutes.

2   Drain the beans; if they're canned, rinse them before draining. Add them to the pot along with the tomatoes and their juices and the stock, rosemary, and thyme. Bring to a boil, then reduce the heat so the soup bubbles steadily; cover and cook, stirring once or twice to break up the tomatoes, until the flavors meld, 15 to 20 minutes.

3   Put a slice of toasted bread in the bottom of each bowl. Raise the heat under the soup to medium-high, add the kale, and cook, stirring occasionally, until the kale is tender and the soup is hot again, 3 to 5 minutes more. Fish out the herb stems if you like, taste and adjust the seasoning, and serve.

VARIATION

SMOOTH AND CREAMY RIBOLLITA This rustic soup turns elegant with only a little extra effort. Just before serving, transfer the soup along with the bread and kale to a blender and carefully puree it until smooth (work in batches if necessary). Return the pureed soup to the stove to reheat until steaming.

MORE IDEAS

Serve the soup over a scoop of brown rice or other whole grain instead of the crouton. • Use chopped green beans instead of the kale.

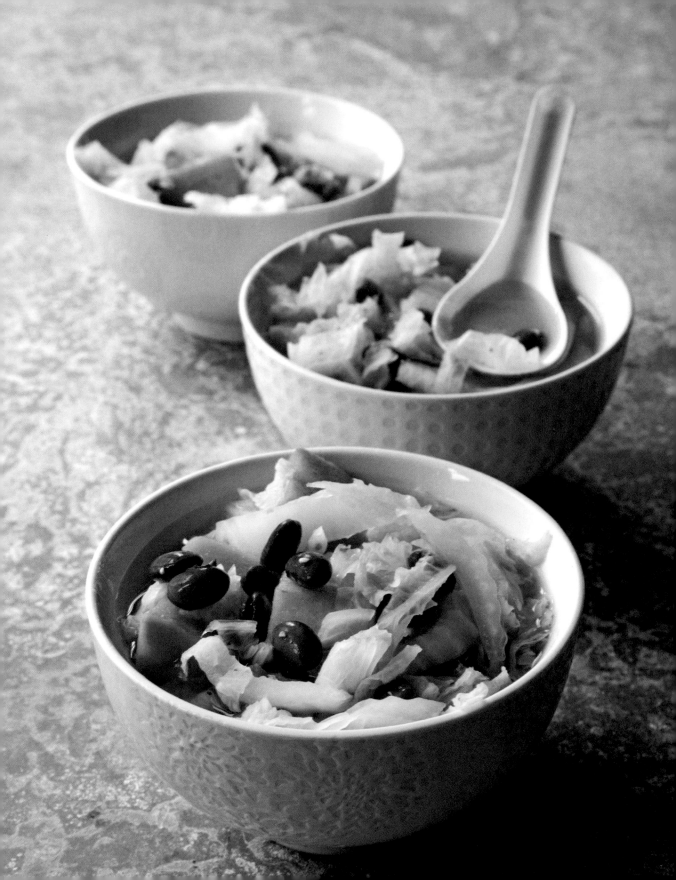

HEARTY MISO SOUP

MAKES 4 servings   **TIME** 40 minutes

For a richly flavored broth in an instant I always turn to miso. Simmering full-flavored vegetables in the liquid first adds even more dimension. If you can't find soybeans, any white or black beans work fine here.

1 pound sweet potatoes, peeled and cut into 2-inch chunks

½ teaspoon salt, plus more to taste

3 cups cooked or canned white or black soybeans (see page 232)

2 pounds napa or savoy cabbage

⅔ cup any miso paste, plus more to taste

¼ cup chopped scallions

1 tablespoon sesame oil

1   Put 8 cups water in a large pot and bring to a boil over medium-high heat. Add the sweet potatoes and salt and cook, stirring once or twice, until they're tender on the outside but still firm at the center, 10 to 15 minutes. If you're using canned beans, rinse and drain them; if homemade beans, just drain them.

2   Add the cabbage and cook, stirring occasionally, until just barely tender, 2 or 3 minutes. Turn off the heat.

3   Put about 1 cup of the cooking liquid in a small bowl and add the miso; whisk until smooth. Stir the miso mixture into the liquid in the pot and turn the heat to medium.

4   Add the beans; stir once or twice and let sit for a minute, still over medium heat, just long enough to heat everything through without letting the soup come to a boil. Taste and adjust the seasoning, adding more miso (whisked with some of the soup) and salt if necessary. Add the scallions, drizzle with the oil, and serve.

MORE IDEAS

Use Asian greens—like bok choy, Chinese broccoli, or mizuna—instead of the cabbage. • Use broccoli, asparagus, zucchini, or green beans instead of the cabbage. • Swap 1 pound tofu cubes for the soybeans. • Try edamame instead of the soybeans.

USING MISO

The easiest way to identify and understand miso—a fermented product made from beans or grains, alone or in combination—is by color. Ranging from mildest (some say sweetest) to most robust, miso is white, yellow, red, and brown. The types are interchangeable in these recipes so use whatever intensity you like best. Some of the better misos have been aged like wine in wooden barrels for years; choose the pastes over super-processed dry or powdered misos for the fullest complexity of flavor. The pastes are worth the investment since they keep for months in the fridge. The most important thing is to avoid boiling miso, which deactivates its beneficial cultures and ruins the taste.

CURRIED CARROT AND LENTIL SOUP

MAKES 4 servings   **TIME** 1 hour, largely unattended

Carrot soup becomes a one-bowl meal when you include a handful of beans in the mix. And if you use lentils it doesn't take any extra time at all—they become tender while the carrots soften.

2 tablespoons vegetable oil

1 onion, chopped

2 tablespoons minced ginger

½ teaspoon salt

¼ teaspoon pepper

1 tablespoon curry powder

1 pound carrots, chopped

¾ cup dried lentils or split peas, washed and picked over

4 cups vegetable stock (see page 246) or water

½ cup coconut milk (reduced-fat is fine)

¼ cup chopped fresh mint or basil, for garnish

1 Put the oil in a large pot over medium-high heat. When it's hot, add the onion and ginger, sprinkle with the salt and pepper, and cook, stirring occasionally, until soft, 3 to 5 minutes.

2 Add the curry powder. Cook, stirring frequently, until fragrant—no more than a minute. Stir in the carrots and lentils. Add the stock and coconut milk. Bring to a boil, then turn the heat down to medium-low so that the soup bubbles gently.

3 Cook, stirring occasionally, until the lentils and vegetables break down, 30 to 40 minutes; add water as necessary to keep the mixture brothy. Taste, adjust the seasoning, garnish, and serve.

MORE IDEAS

For a bit of sweetness, add 1 cup chopped dried apricots or peaches along with the lentils and carrots in Step 2. • Go green; toss in 2 (or more) cups chopped kale, collards, or spinach about 5 minutes before the soup is done cooking. • Instead of the carrots, try parsnips, celery root, or winter or summer squash.

RHUBARB AND RED LENTIL SOUP

MAKES 4 servings   TIME 45 minutes, largely unattended

Red lentils (actually, they're bright orange) cook up rich and creamy in a
flash. The tart fruit here provides the perfect balance while melting away
to almost nothing. While I like this as a soup, you can also serve it as
you would any dal, over rice or cooked vegetables, or use it as a sauce for
meat, chicken, or fish.

3 tablespoons vegetable oil

1 onion, chopped

1 tablespoon minced garlic

2 tablespoons minced
ginger

1 teaspoon salt

½ teaspoon pepper

4 cardamom pods

1 tablespoon mustard
seeds

2 cloves

3 or 4 rhubarb stalks,
strings removed, chopped

1 cup dried red lentils,
rinsed

1 quart vegetable stock (see
page 246) or water

¼ cup chopped fresh
cilantro, for garnish

1 Put the oil in a large pot over medium-high heat. When it's hot, add
the onion and cook, stirring occasionally, until soft, 3 to 5 minutes. Add
the garlic and ginger and cook for another minute. Sprinkle with the salt
and pepper.

2 Add the cardamom pods, mustard seeds, and cloves. Cook and stir
until fragrant, about 30 seconds. Stir in the rhubarb and lentils. Add the
stock and bring to a boil; turn the heat down so the soup bubbles gently
but steadily.

3 Cover the pot and cook, stirring occasionally, until the lentils and
vegetables become almost smooth, 30 to 35 minutes; add water as
necessary to keep the mixture brothy. Taste, adjust the seasoning, fish
out the whole spices if you like, and serve, garnished with the cilantro.

MORE IDEAS

If you can't find red lentils easily, you can make this soup with brown or green
lentils instead. • Some other fruits to try instead of the rhubarb are peaches,
plums, apricots, or tomatoes (they're a fruit, remember!).

ORANGE SOUP WITH BLACK SALSA

MAKES 4 servings   **TIME** About 1 hour

Squash soup, which is wonderfully smooth and rich, becomes bolder
and heartier with the addition of beans. Both components can be made
ahead and stored in individual containers to be assembled for quick
midweek meals.

1 cup cooked or canned
black beans (see page 232)

2 tomatoes, chopped

1 small red onion, chopped

1 fresh hot chile (like
jalapeño), seeded and
minced

½ cup chopped fresh
cilantro

2 tablespoons lime juice

1 teaspoon salt

1 teaspoon pepper

3 tablespoons olive oil

1 large onion, chopped

2 tablespoons minced garlic

1½ pounds winter squash
(like butternut or pumpkin),
cut into cubes

2 teaspoons chili powder

1 teaspoon cumin

6 cups vegetable stock (see
page 246) or water

1   Drain the beans; if they're canned, rinse them before draining.
Combine the tomatoes, onion, chile, beans, cilantro, lime juice, and half
the salt and pepper in a bowl. Stir and then let the salsa sit while the
soup simmers (or you can make it up to 1 day in advance and refrigerate
until you're ready to make the soup).

2   Put the olive oil in a large pot over medium-high heat. When it's
hot, add the onion and garlic, and cook, stirring occasionally, until soft,
3 to 5 minutes. Add the squash, chili powder, cumin, and remaining
½ teaspoon salt and pepper. Cook, stirring constantly, until fragrant,
about 1 minute.

3   Add the vegetable stock, bring to a boil, and reduce the heat so
the soup bubbles gently. Cover and cook, stirring once in a while until
squash is tender and falling apart, 20 to 25 minutes.

4   Transfer the soup to a blender (working in batches if necessary) or
use an immersion blender to carefully puree the soup. Reheat it until
just bubbling, adding more water if necessary. Top each bowl of soup
with some black bean salsa, and serve.

VARIATION

SQUASH SOUP WITH APPLE SALSA Perfect in winter. For the salsa,
use green apples instead of the tomatoes. If you'd like to change the
seasoning, use cinnamon instead of cumin.

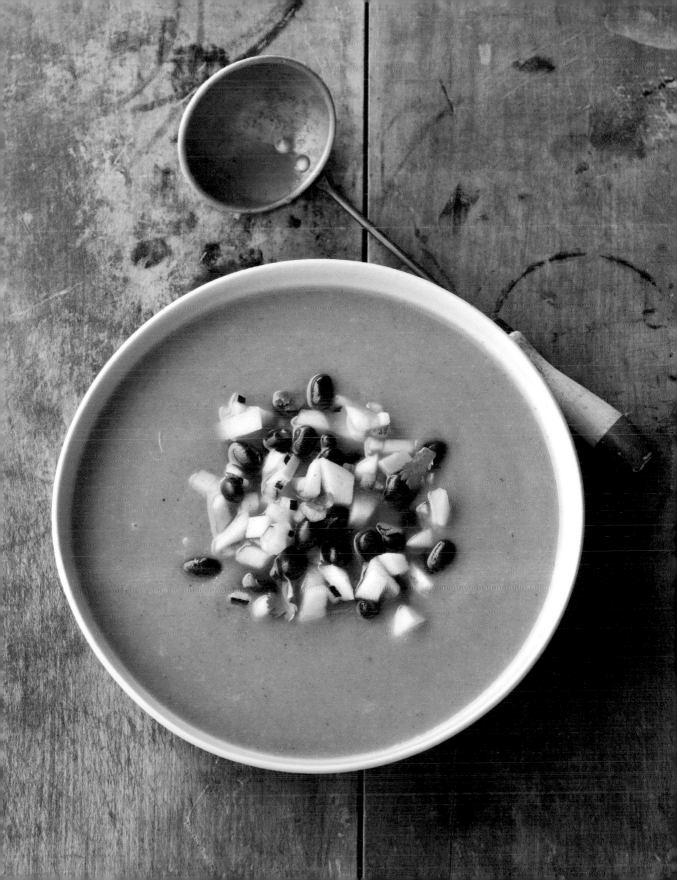

CREAMY TOMATO SOUP

MAKES **4 servings**   TIME **45 minutes**

If there ever was an iconic soup, this is it: comforting, satisfying, and always delicious. Eat it with some toasted, crusty bread on the side for dipping, or half a griddled peanut butter sandwich. Awesome. Really.

2 tablespoons olive oil

1 large onion, halved and thinly sliced

1 carrot, chopped

1 celery stalk, chopped

1 tablespoon minced garlic

½ teaspoon salt

¼ teaspoon pepper

2 tablespoons tomato paste

2 fresh thyme sprigs, or 1 teaspoon dried

2 pounds tomatoes, chopped, or one 28-ounce can diced tomatoes, including the juice

2 cups tomato juice or water

12 ounces silken tofu (1½ cups)

1 cup chopped fresh basil leaves, for garnish

1 Put the oil in a large pot over medium heat. When it's hot, add the onion, carrot, celery, and garlic; sprinkle with the salt and pepper, and cook, stirring, until the vegetables soften, 5 to 10 minutes. Add the tomato paste and continue to cook, stirring, until the paste is distributed and begins to darken (don't let it burn), 1 or 2 minutes.

2 Strip the thyme leaves from the stems and add them to the pot along with the tomatoes and tomato juice or water. Bring to a boil, then adjust the heat so the mixture bubbles gently but steadily. Cook, stirring occasionally, until the tomatoes break down, 10 to 15 minutes.

3 Add the tofu and cook, stirring and breaking it up with the spoon for another minute. If the soup is too thick, add more water, ¼ cup at a time. If it's too thin, continue to cook until it thickens and reduces slightly (this will also intensify the flavors).

4 Transfer the soup to a blender (working in batches if necessary) or use an immersion blender to carefully puree the soup. Reheat it until just bubbling, adding more water if necessary to thin it. Taste and adjust the seasoning and serve, garnished with the basil.

VARIATION

BUTTERNUT SQUASH SOUP Swap cubed squash for tomatoes and omit the tomato paste. Use water or vegetable stock instead of tomato juice. In Step 2, cook the squash until soft, 15 to 20 minutes, before blending. Drizzle with balsamic vinegar before garnishing if you'd like.

MORE IDEAS

This is essentially cream of anything soup: Chop a vegetable (or vegetables) and cook with aromatics as described in Step 2. You're going to have to adjust the cooking time to accommodate firmer and more tender vegetables and add enough water or stock to make it "soupy," but use the techniques as described and you'll do fine.

RED SOUP

MAKES **4 servings**   TIME **45 minutes**

Borscht, beefed up with beans and even more vegetables, is earthy, herba-ceous, bright-tasting . . . and the color can't be beat.

3 cups cooked or canned kidney beans

2 tablespoons olive oil

1 large red onion, chopped

1 teaspoon salt

½ teaspoon pepper

1½ pounds beets, chopped

½ head red cabbage, chopped

6 cups vegetable stock (see page 246) or water

1 tablespoon cider vinegar

¼ cup chopped fresh dill, or 2 teaspoons dried

1 If you're using canned beans, rinse and drain them; if you're using homemade beans, drain them, reserving the cooking liquid to replace some of the vegetable stock.

2 Put the oil in a large pot over medium-high heat. Add the onion, sprinkle with salt and pepper, and cook, stirring occasionally, until soft, 2 or 3 minutes. Turn the heat to medium-low and continue cooking, stirring occasionally, until very tender, 10 to 15 minutes more.

3 Add the beets and cabbage, stirring to coat in the oil. Add the stock and beans and bring to a boil, then lower the heat so the soup bubbles gently but steadily. Cover and cook, stirring once or twice, until the vegetables are starting to melt away, 15 to 20 minutes. Stir in the vinegar and dill. Taste and adjust the seasoning, and serve.

VARIATIONS

WHITE SOUP Substitute white onion, turnips, green cabbage, and navy beans for the red onion, beets, red cabbage, and kidney beans.

ESCAROLE AND WHITE BEAN SOUP Make a completely different classic soup simply by changing ingredients. Skip the beets. Substitute 2 leeks for the onion, 2 heads of escarole for the cabbage, and cannellini for the kidney beans. Use fresh parsley instead of dill.

MORE IDEAS

Stir in diced red or sweet potatoes along with the beets. • Put a scoop of brown rice or other whole grain in the middle of the bowl after serving. • Top the soup with whole wheat croutons or breadcrumbs. • Garnish with chopped hazelnuts.

GRAINS MARINARA

MAKES 4 servings   **TIME** 10 to 20 minutes with cooked grains

This recipe makes a strong case for why you should always have cooked grains in your refrigerator: It's unbelievably good, and you'll find yourself returning to it constantly as a springboard for quick one-skillet lunches. You decide if you want the tomatoes almost raw, coddled, or saucy. You can scale it down for one or two servings quite easily.

2 tablespoons olive oil

1 small onion, chopped

1 tablespoon minced garlic

1 teaspoon salt

½ teaspoon pepper

1½ pounds Roma (plum) tomatoes, chopped

4 cups any cooked grain, like brown rice, bulgur quinoa, farro, wheat berries, or oat groats

½ cup chopped fresh basil, for garnish

1   Put the olive oil in a large skillet over medium-high heat. When it's hot, add the onion and garlic, sprinkle with the salt and pepper, and cook, stirring occasionally, until the vegetables soften a bit, 2 or 3 minutes.

2   Add the tomatoes, and once they start to cook, stir frequently until they reach the doneness you want: 2 or 3 minutes for just warm, 3 to 5 minutes for tender but intact, and up to 10 minutes for them to break down and make a sauce.

3   Add the grain, stirring and breaking it up with the back of a spoon or a fork until evenly distributed and heated through. Taste and adjust the seasoning and serve, garnished with the basil.

VARIATIONS

GRAINS SALSA ROJO Spicier, for sure. Use Cooked Red Salsa (page 239 or store-bought, if you must) instead of the tomato sauce; you'll need 2 to 3 cups. Heat it until it bubbles steadily, then skip to Step 3.

GRAINS SALSA VERDE Gorgeous green color and bright, tangy flavor. Use Cooked Green Salsa (page 239 or store-bought, if you must) instead of the tomato sauce; you'll need 2 to 3 cups. Heat it until it bubbles steadily, then skip to Step 3.

MORE IDEAS

Add cooked vegetables at will: Heat them in the tomatoes for a minute, just before stirring in the grains. • If you have leftover tomato sauce in the fridge, all the better. Warm at least ½ cup per serving before adding the grains. • For a creamier texture, try using porridge for the cooked grains. Polenta, grits, cracked wheat, or rolled or steel-cut oats will be soupier but equally delicious. • Go ahead and use canned tomatoes here. Figure one 28-ounce can. • If you don't have fresh basil, try ¼ cup chopped fresh parsley, mint, dill, or cilantro; or 1 tablespoon chopped fresh oregano, thyme, or rosemary. • And if you don't have any fresh herbs, add 1 teaspoon dried oregano or thyme (or curry powder for an interesting twist) to the tomatoes in Step 2.

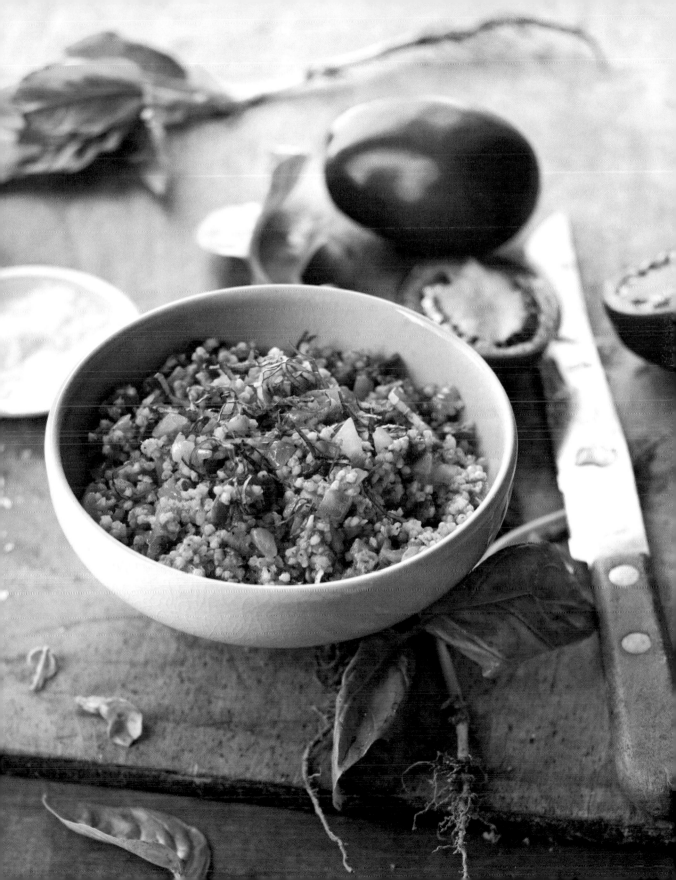

SPAGHETTI WITH BEAN BOLOGNESE

MAKES 4 servings   TIME 30 minutes

Bolognese sans meat and dairy is still pretty great, as hearty and thick as the original. And as with any good sauce, you'll want to eat it all the time—spooned over toast, rice or other grains, or steamed greens—so be smart and make a double recipe. The additional effort is negligible.

3 cups cooked or canned pinto or kidney beans (see page 232)

3 tablespoons olive oil

1 onion, chopped

1 carrot, chopped

1 zucchini, chopped

1 red bell pepper, chopped

2 tablespoons minced garlic

½ teaspoon salt

½ teaspoon pepper

One 28-ounce can whole Roma (plum) tomatoes

8 ounces whole wheat spaghetti

1 cup chopped fresh basil

1 If you're using canned beans, rinse and drain them; if you cooked the beans yourself, drain them, reserving the cooking liquid. Put the oil in a large pot over medium heat. When it's hot, add the onion, carrot, zucchini, bell pepper, and garlic. Sprinkle with the salt and pepper and cook, stirring occasionally, until the vegetables soften, 5 to 10 minutes.

2 Add the tomatoes and beans to the pot and bring to a boil, then adjust the heat so the mixture bubbles gently but steadily. Cook, stirring once in a while to break up the tomatoes, until the beans are quite tender and the tomato sauce is slightly thickened, 15 to 20 minutes.

3 Bring a large pot of water to a boil and salt it. Cook the pasta until it's tender but not mushy (start tasting after 5 minutes), then drain, reserving some of the cooking liquid. Toss the pasta with the sauce and the basil, adding enough reserved pasta cooking water (or bean cooking liquid) to keep it moist. Taste, adjust the seasoning, and serve.

VARIATION

TOFU TOMATO SAUCE OVER SPAGHETTI OR BROWN RICE Substitute 1½ pounds tofu for the beans, and if you'd like, make brown rice instead of the spaghetti (see page 230). Crumble it into the pot after cooking the vegetables in Step 1.

MORE IDEAS

Instead of using the zucchini and pepper here, try mushrooms, fennel, or escarole. • Make this with fresh tomatoes: You'll need about 2 pounds of whichever kind you like as long as they're super ripe. I don't bother to peel and seed them, though you certainly can if you're feeling ambitious. • Instead of red beans, use frozen fava or lima beans, black-eyed peas, black beans, or cannellini. • If you don't have fresh basil handy, try half the amount of fresh parsley or 1 tablespoon fresh oregano. Or add 1 teaspoon dried oregano to the vegetables as they cook. • Use any pasta shape you like. • Skip the beans and serve the sauce and pasta with Eggplant Meatballs (page 124).

SEAWEED SOBA

MAKES 4 servings **TIME** 30 minutes

Something wonderful happens when you use the liquid from cooking vegetables to boil noodles: One flavors the other. Add the brininess of kombu—kelp, in English—and you have a quick and somewhat miraculous one-dish meal. If you've never worked with seaweed before, this simple preparation has a subtle taste and is a perfect introduction.

½ ounce dried kombu (3 or 4 large pieces or 2 sheets); or 6 cups vegetable stock (see page 246)

2 teaspoons salt

12 ounces winter squash (like kabocha or pumpkin), peeled and seeded

8 ounces mushrooms (like shiitake, button, or cremini), sliced

8 ounces soba noodles

2 tablespoons soy sauce

1 tablespoon mirin

½ cup chopped scallions, for garnish

1 tablespoon sesame oil

1 Put 6 cups water in a medium saucepan over high heat. When it just starts to bubble, turn off the heat and add the kombu; cover and let sit 15 minutes. (Or heat the stock instead.)

2 Bring a large pot of water to a boil and add the salt. Chop the squash into 1-inch chunks; you should have about 2 cups. Once the water has come to a boil, add the squash and cook, stirring occasionally, until tender, 8 to 10 minutes. Transfer to a bowl using a slotted spoon. Add the mushrooms and cook 1 minute, add them to the bowl with the squash, and return the water to a boil. Add the noodles and cook, stirring once or twice and adjusting the heat so the water bubbles steadily until just barely tender, 3 to 5 minutes. Drain the noodles, reserving 1 cup of the cooking liquid, and return the noodles and vegetables to the pot, off heat.

3 Lift the kombu from the soaking liquid and cut into thin strips. Add sliced kombu and its soaking liquid to the noodles and vegetables in the pot along with the soy sauce and mirin. Warm the noodles and broth over medium heat, stirring once or twice, adding some reserved cooking liquid if you'd like, and adjusting the heat so the broth doesn't boil. Taste and adjust the seasoning, test a noodle for doneness, and serve, garnished with the scallions and drizzled with the sesame oil.

VARIATIONS

SOBA WITH SUMMER SQUASH, MUSHROOMS, AND SEA GREENS Use summer squash instead of winter squash; pattypan is the best for this but yellow squash or zucchini works well, too. Adjust the time in Step 2 so that the squash only cooks for 2 or 3 minutes before removing and proceeding with the recipe.

SOBA WITH DAIKON, MUSHROOMS, AND SEA GREENS Substitute daikon for the squash. Peel and cut it into 1-inch chunks. Add 1 tablespoon minced ginger to the pot with the daikon in Step 2.

TOFU STEAKS WITH COLD NOODLES

MAKES 4 servings   **TIME** 30 minutes

Making sesame noodles—the iconic restaurant dish—yourself is not only better, it allows you to use fewer noodles and more vegetables, which are the best, most refreshing part. Frozen edamame are great here—as they thaw they'll help chill the salad. And one final tip: Serving the noodles on top of tofu steaks is easy and impressive; but if you want more crunch throughout, see the first variation.

1½ teaspoons salt

3 tablespoons tahini

2 teaspoons rice vinegar

1 tablespoon soy sauce

1 teaspoon sesame oil

½ teaspoon pepper

1 cucumber, peeled, seeded, and grated

1 red bell pepper, thinly sliced

1 cup chopped scallions

1½ cups shelled fresh or frozen edamame

2 tablespoons vegetable oil

1 pound firm tofu (1 block), cut lengthwise into 4 slices

8 ounces soba noodles

¼ cup chopped fresh cilantro, for garnish

1 tablespoon sesame seeds, for garnish

1 Bring a large pot of water to a boil and add 1 teaspoon salt. Put the tahini in a large bowl with the vinegar, soy sauce, sesame oil, ¼ teaspoon each of salt and pepper. Add ¼ cup water and whisk until smooth. Squeeze as much liquid as you can from the grated cucumber and add it to the bowl with the dressing, along with the bell pepper, scallions, and edamame.

2 Put the vegetable oil in a large skillet (preferably cast-iron or non-stick) over medium-high heat. When it's hot, add the tofu and sprinkle with the remaining ¼ teaspoon salt and ¼ teaspoon pepper. Cook the steaks, undisturbed, until they're browned and release easily from the pan, 3 to 5 minutes. Turn and repeat with the other side. Transfer the steaks to plates.

3 Once the water has come to a boil, add the noodles and cook until tender but not mushy, 4 to 5 minutes. Drain them and rinse under cold running water and add them to the dressing and vegetables; toss with tongs until all the ingredients are evenly distributed. (The salad and tofu can both be made up to several hours ahead and refrigerated.) Taste and adjust the seasoning, toss again, and serve the noodles atop the tofu, garnished with the cilantro and sesame seeds.

VARIATIONS

COLD SESAME NOODLES WITH CRISP TOFU CUBES Instead of four thick slices, cut the tofu into 1-inch cubes. Cook as directed in Step 2, only after they start to release from the pan, stir-fry them, tossing occasionally and scraping up any browned bits with a spatula, until they're crisp all over, another 3 to 5 minutes. Toss the tofu cubes with the noodles and dressing in Step 3.

COLD SESAME NOODLES WITH EDAMAME Omit the tofu and vegetable oil and skip Step 2. Increase the amount of edamame to 3 cups.

Other vegetables to add or substitute in this dish are thin ribbons of a mild cabbage like napa or savoy or Asian greens like bok choy or mizuna, bean sprouts, or sliced celery or daikon radish. • Instead of edamame, use frozen lima beans or fava beans. • Replace the tahini with peanut or cashew butter and call this—what else?—Peanut or Cashew Noodles. • For an alternative to noodles, try brown rice or whole wheat spaghetti. Increase the cooking time by a couple minutes and check frequently to avoid overcooking. • Lemon or lime juice is a good stand-in for the rice vinegar.

BUYING AND STORING TOFU

People in China have been eating tofu—known there as *dofu*—for at least 2,000 years, though its exact date of origin hasn't been pinpointed. I'm serious when I say that tofu is a cheese made from soybeans: Once the milk is extracted, a coagulant breaks the liquid into curds and whey, which are then separated so that the solids can be shaped into blocks.

There are enough kinds of tofu to make your head spin, but for the purposes of recipes in this book they fall into two categories: *firm* (usually packed in water and sold in the refrigerator case) and *silken* (usually packed in aseptic boxes and stored at room temperature). To make firm tofu, the soymilk solids are separated and pressed into molds to form blocks that can be sliced, cubed, or crumbled or mashed like feta. For silken tofu, the liquid isn't drained off; instead it's formed under pressure, resulting in a custard-like smooth texture.

Both types are available in various degrees of firmness, but I've never found it matters much. Generally I just buy firm or extra-firm of both kinds, since I'm always trying to remove moisture anyway. If you want more delicate smoothies, you might consider a soft silken tofu, but that's nuanced choice. Blocks of firm tofu weigh between 14 and 16 ounces; boxes of silken tofu usually weigh 12 ounces. Once you open tofu, you've got to use it fairly quickly; it's best within a couple days.

CAPONATA MIXED RICE

MAKES 4 servings   TIME 30 minutes

Caponata is an 18th-century Mediterranean eggplant-based relish that's generally served cold as an antipasto on toast or crackers. Assumed to be Sicilian, the recipe might actually come from Spain, where some say it was served like gazpacho. Either way, it's great. Here, I mix the classic ingredients into a risottolike dish based on brown rice.

3 tablespoons olive oil

1 onion, chopped

1 cup short-grain brown rice

1 tablespoon minced garlic

½ teaspoon salt

½ teaspoon black pepper

1½ pounds tomatoes, chopped

1 pound eggplant, peeled if you like, cubed

2 tablespoons drained capers

½ cup chopped fresh parsley

2 tablespoons balsamic vinegar

1 Put the oil in a large pot over medium heat. When it's hot, add the onion and cook, stirring occasionally, until translucent, 2 to 3 minutes. Add the rice and garlic, sprinkle with the salt and pepper, and continue to cook, stirring occasionally, until the rice is shiny and smells toasty, another 1 or 2 minutes. Add enough water to cover by about ½ inch.

2 Bring to a boil, then lower the heat so that it bubbles gently. Cook, stirring occasionally, until the rice just starts to become tender, 10 to 15 minutes. Add the tomatoes and eggplant and continue to cook, stirring occasionally, until the tomatoes break down and the eggplant softens, 5 to 10 minutes more. Add more water if needed to keep the mixture a little soupy.

3 Continue to cook, stirring occasionally until the mixture is no longer soupy but not yet dry. Test a kernel of rice: It should be tender outside but still retain some bite at the core; it might take another 5 to 10 minutes to reach this point.

4 Stir in the capers, parsley, and vinegar. Taste and adjust the seasoning and serve.

VARIATIONS

BROCCOLI-TOMATO MIXED RICE For those who don't like eggplant, substitute broccoli; break it into small florets and slice the stalks before adding it to the rice in Step 2.

CAULIFLOWER-TOMATO MIXED RICE Same deal as with broccoli, only it will take a little longer to cook.

MORE IDEAS

Top the rice with toasted pine nuts for added crunch. • Add ¼ cup currants or raisins when you add the capers in Step 3. • Use ¼ cup chopped black olives instead of the capers. Kalamata or dry-cured work best here. • Try fresh basil, mint, or dill instead of the parsley.

EDAMAME FRIED RICE

MAKES 4 servings   TIME 30 minutes with cooked rice

I love variations on this theme for dinner, lunch, and even breakfast. You will too, especially if you consider the recipe here as a blueprint, then slot in substitutions freely with any leftover cooked vegetables or grains.

3 tablespoons vegetable oil

1 onion, chopped

1 small head broccoli, chopped

½ teaspoon salt

2 cups edamame (frozen is fine)

1 large carrot, grated

1 cup bean sprouts

1 tablespoon minced garlic

1 tablespoon minced ginger

3 cups cooked brown rice, any kind (see page 230)

1 tablespoon soy sauce, plus more to taste

1 tablespoon sesame oil

¼ teaspoon pepper

½ cup chopped scallions

¼ cup chopped fresh cilantro, for garnish

1 Put 1 tablespoon of the oil in a large skillet over high heat. When it's hot, add the onion, broccoli, and ¼ teaspoon of the salt and cook, stirring occasionally, until they soften and begin to brown, 3 to 5 minutes. Lower the heat if the mixture threatens to scorch. Transfer the vegetables to a large bowl with a slotted spoon.

2 Return the pan to the heat with another 1 tablespoon oil. Add the edamame, carrot, and bean sprouts along with ¼ cup water and the remaining ¼ teaspoon salt; cook, shaking the skillet until the water bubbles away, 1 or 2 minutes. Add to the bowl with the vegetables.

3 Put the remaining 1 tablespoon oil in the skillet and return the pan to the heat; add the garlic and ginger. About 15 seconds later, begin to scatter the rice into the pan a bit at a time, breaking up any clumps with your fingers. Cook, undisturbed, until you hear the rice sizzle and smell it toasting (but not burning).

4 Return the edamame and vegetables to the pan and stir quickly to integrate. Add more water, 2 tablespoons at a time, to help release any browned bits from the bottom of the pan and cook, stirring, for about 1 minute. Add the soy sauce, sesame oil, and pepper, then taste and adjust the seasoning if necessary. Turn off the heat, stir in the scallions, garnish with the cilantro, and serve.

VARIATION

FRIED RICE WITH CASHEWS AND PINEAPPLE Use 2 cups chopped fresh pineapple instead of the broccoli and increase the bean sprouts to 2 cups. Add ½ cup cashews with the garlic and ginger in Step 3. Add 1 tomato, chopped, with the scallions if you like.

MORE IDEAS

The list of possible additions or substitutions is long. Here's a start: bell peppers, mushrooms, water chestnuts, snow peas, snap peas, green beans spinach, bok choy, cabbage. • Swap cubes of smoked tofu or any of the basic tofu preparations on pages 240–41. • Use other cooked, canned, or frozen beans; limas, black beans, or chickpeas hold up best. • Instead of rice, try cooked quinoa, bulgur, wheat berries, or farro. • Add herbs: basil (especially Thai), mint, or lemongrass are my favorites in fried rice.

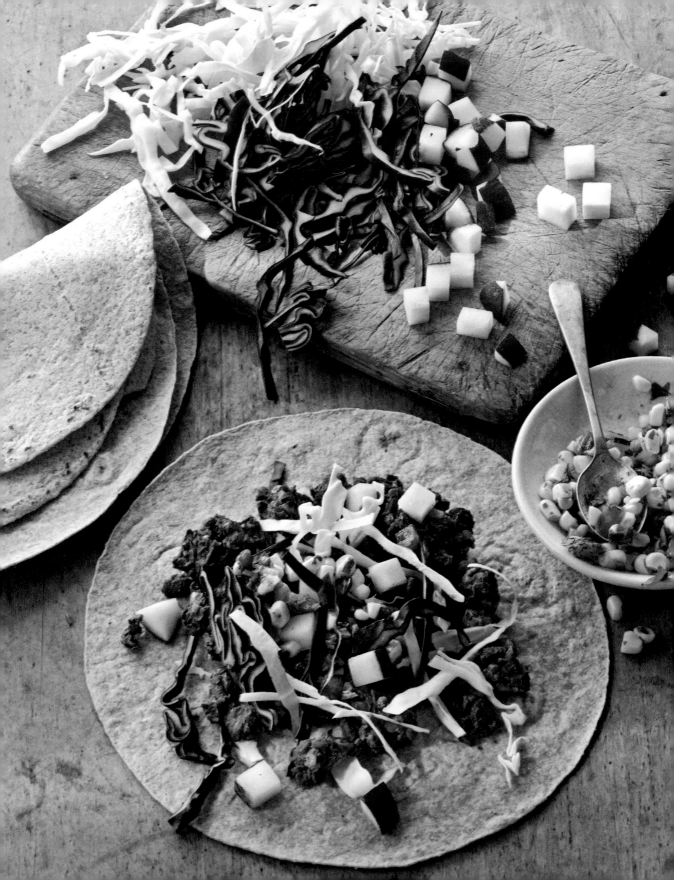

FULLY LOADED BEAN BURRITOS

MAKES 4 servings   TIME 30 minutes

At its best, a jam-packed burrito can take you halfway through the day without weighing you down. The key is to focus on beans and vegetables—and be willing to eat whatever falls out of the tortilla with a fork (or, of course, your fingers).

Four 8-inch whole wheat flour tortillas

2 tablespoons olive oil

1 red onion, chopped

1 tablespoon minced garlic

1 tablespoon chili powder

½ teaspoon salt

¼ teaspoon pepper

2 cups cooked or canned black beans (see page 232)

2 cups shredded red or green cabbage

4 radishes, chopped

1 cup (or more) Pico de Gallo (page 236) or Salsa (page 239)

1 Heat the oven to 300°F. Stack the tortillas and roll them up in a sheet of foil. Put them in the oven to warm while you cook the filling.

2 Put the oil in a large skillet over medium heat. When it's hot, add the onion and garlic and cook, stirring occasionally, until soft, 3 to 5 minutes. Sprinkle with the chili powder, salt, and pepper.

3 Drain the beans; if they're canned, rinse them also. Add the beans to the skillet; mash them up a bit with a fork or potato masher and add a spoonful of water if the mixture seems dry. Taste and adjust the seasoning and remove from the heat.

4 To roll the burritos, lay a tortilla on a flat surface and put one-fourth of the filling on the third closest to you. Top with some cabbage, radishes, and pico de gallo. Fold the tortilla over from the bottom to cover the fillings, then fold in the two sides to enclose it fully; finish rolling, then put the burrito seam side down on a plate. Repeat to make three more burritos. Serve with more pico de gallo on the side if you like.

VARIATIONS

HOT AND SMOKY BLACK BEAN BURRITOS Beware—you're cranking up the heat here. Add 1 chopped jalapeño and 1 or 2 chopped chipotle chiles (with some of their adobo if you'd like) to the black beans in Step 2.

SPANISH-STYLE BURRITO Change the flavor profile in a flash by using chickpeas instead of the black beans, and smoked paprika instead of the chili powder.

CAULIFLOWER ROMESCO

MAKES 4 servings   **TIME** About 30 minutes

Nuts, garlic, and tomatoes are the main components of a traditional Catalan romesco sauce, but beyond that there's a lot of elbow room for variation, including what you serve it with. It's perfect with other fresh or roasted vegetables, on toast, stirred into rice, or served with simply cooked tofu, chicken, fish, lamb or pork chops, or steak.

1½ pounds cauliflower, separated into large florets

3 tablespoons olive oil

½ teaspoon salt

¼ teaspoon pepper

1 pound Roma (plum) tomatoes, halved

½ cup almonds

2 tablespoons chopped garlic

1 tablespoon sherry or red wine vinegar, or more to taste

¼ cup chopped fresh parsley

1 Heat the oven to 450°F. Put the cauliflower in a roasting pan or rimmed baking sheet, drizzle with 1 tablespoon oil, sprinkle with half the salt and pepper, and toss to distribute. Put the tomatoes, almonds, and garlic in another pan and repeat with the remaining 2 tablespoons oil, ¼ teaspoon salt, and ⅛ teaspoon pepper.

2 Transfer both pans to the oven and roast, stirring once or twice, until the vegetables are tender and charred in places. The tomato mixture will be ready first, in 5 to 10 minutes; transfer it and any juices to a blender or food processor. Leave the cauliflower in the oven until it's tender, another 15 to 20 minutes.

3 Add the vinegar to the blender with the tomatoes, and pulse until the sauce is as coarse or as smooth as you like; to thin it, add water, 1 tablespoon at a time as you work. Transfer the romesco to a small pot to warm over medium heat if you'd like. Taste and adjust the seasoning, spoon over the cauliflower, garnish, and serve.

VARIATION

CAULIFLOWER ROMESCO SOUP Terrific, and has only one more step. Heat 4 cups vegetable stock in a large pot until bubbling steadily. After completing the recipe, puree the cauliflower with the romesco and stir the mixture into the stock until it's thick and creamy.

MORE IDEAS

Add some heat to the romesco by roasting 1 or more cored jalapeños or other hot chiles with the tomatoes. • Use hazelnuts or pecans instead of the almonds. • Use Cauliflower Romesco as a sauce to toss with any shape cooked pasta; mash it up first as little or as much as you like.

CURRIED SPINACH AND TOFU

MAKES 4 servings   TIME 30 minutes

Take saag paneer—the classic Indian dish of fresh cheese and pureed spinach—and substitute both firm and silken tofu for the dairy, and bingo: vegan saag paneer. And it's terrific. For a completely different approach, try the tomato-chickpea variation.

3 tablespoons vegetable oil

1 small red onion, halved and sliced

2 tablespoons minced ginger

8 ounces silken tofu (about 1 cup)

2 tablespoons curry powder or garam masala

1 teaspoon salt

½ teaspoon pepper

1½ pounds spinach, rinsed well and trimmed

1 pound firm tofu (1 block), cut into 1-inch cubes

2 lemons, cut into wedges for serving

1 Put the oil in a large pot over medium heat. Add the onion and ginger and cook, stirring frequently, until the vegetables soften and begin to turn golden, 5 to 10 minutes. Put the silken tofu in a small bowl and whisk until smooth. (It will go through an awkward "broken" stage— just keep whisking until the mixture emulsifies.)

2 Add the curry powder, salt, and pepper to the onion mixture and cook, stirring constantly, until fragrant, about 1 minute. Start adding the spinach a handful at a time, until the pan is full. Stir frequently and adjust the heat as necessary so the spinach softens but doesn't burn; when there's room in the skillet, add more spinach and stir, repeating until all the spinach is used. Then cook, stirring occasionally, until the pan is almost dry, just another 1 or 2 minutes.

3 Add the silken tofu and cook, stirring constantly and adjusting the heat as necessary, until the mixture bubbles gently but steadily. Add the firm tofu and cover. Cook, stirring once or twice, until the cubes are heated through, 2 to 3 minutes. Taste and adjust the seasoning and serve with the lemon wedges.

VARIATION

CURRIED SPINACH WITH TOMATOES AND CHICKPEAS Perfect in summer when tomatoes are at their best, but good with canned tomatoes too. Skip the tofus and substitute 3 cups chopped tomatoes for the silken tofu and 3 cups drained and rinsed chickpeas for the firm. In Step 2, add the tomatoes as soon as all the spinach is in the pan. Then add the chickpeas instead of the cubes in Step 3 and cook until just heated through, 2 to 3 minutes.

MORE IDEAS

Use chopped cabbage, chard, or Brussels sprouts instead of the spinach.
• Skip the firm tofu cubes (but keep the silken tofu) and try finishing the dish with ½ cup chopped pistachios.

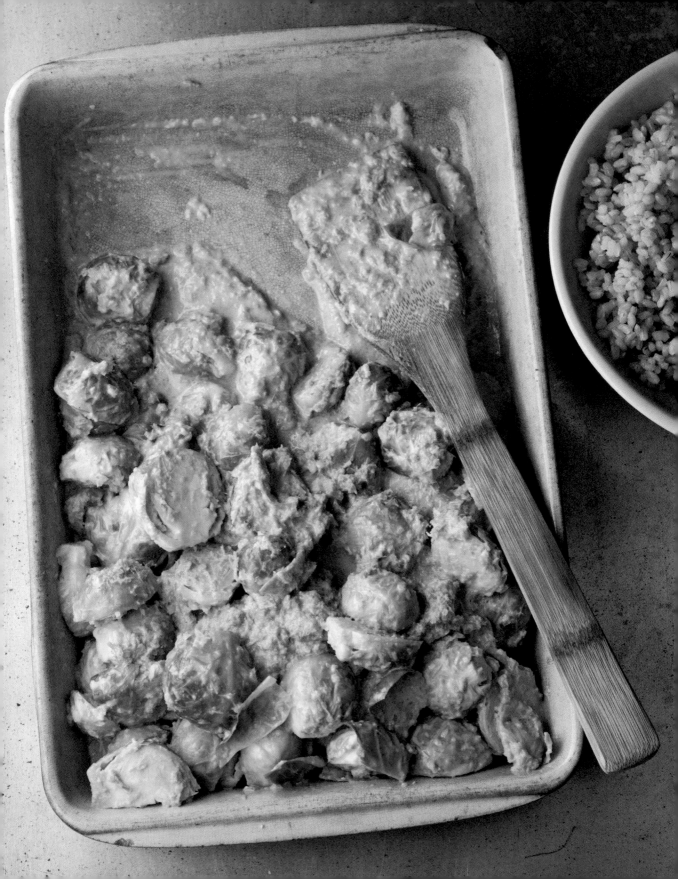

SLOW-COOKED BRUSSELS SPROUTS WITH LEMONGRASS

MAKES 4 servings   TIME About 1 hour

To intensely flavor vegetables I sometimes use the Malaysian technique of boiling down coconut milk until all that remains is coconut oil and milk solids. The resulting dish is called *rendang*, which usually contains meat but is fantastic for Brussels sprouts (and more; see the variation and ideas that follow) since the vegetables slow-cook before browning. Serve over brown rice, topped with pickled vegetables (see page 138).

2 thick fresh lemongrass stalks

2 limes

5 small shallots or 3 large shallots, cut into chunks

3 garlic cloves, smashed

1½ teaspoons ground turmeric

2-inch piece ginger, peeled and cut into chunks

1 fresh chile (like Thai or jalapeño), cut into chunks

1 cup coconut milk (reduced-fat is fine)

1 cup unsweetened plain non-dairy milk, like oat or rice

1½ pounds Brussels sprouts, trimmed and halved

1 Remove the tough parts of the lemongrass stalks and discard; chop the tender and aromatic centers. Zest one lime and cut the other into wedges. Combine the lemongrass, shallots, garlic, turmeric, ginger, chile, and lime zest in a small food processor or coffee grinder (or use a mortar and pestle). Pulse (or mash) until the mixture forms a paste, adding a teaspoon of water if necessary.

2 Put the paste in a deep skillet over medium heat. Stir and cook until fragrant, just 1 or 2 minutes, then add both milks. Stir to combine and adjust the heat so the mixture bubbles gently but steadily: Cook, uncovered and stirring once in a while, until the liquid is reduced by half, 20 to 30 minutes.

3 Add the Brussels sprouts and adjust the heat so the mixture barely bubbles. Cook, uncovered and stirring infrequently, until the sprouts are tender throughout and the pan is dry, 30 to 35 minutes. Taste and adjust the seasoning, then serve garnished with the lime wedges.

VARIATION

SLOW-COOKED EGGPLANT WITH CURRY Substitute eggplant for the Brussels sprouts; cut them into 1-inch cubes. Instead of the lemongrass and turmeric, use 1 tablespoon curry powder and cook it in the hot oil with the other ingredients as described in Step 2.

MORE IDEAS

All sorts of other vegetables work well in this recipe. Try chunks of carrots, red or green cabbage, cauliflower, broccoli, green beans, or potatoes with the seasoning of either the main recipe or the variation.

TERIYAKI TEMPEH WITH BOK CHOY

MAKES 4 servings   TIME 30 minutes

The contrast of crisp and tangy tempeh—a fermented cake of soybeans
and sometimes grains—silky braised bok choy, and familiar, sweet-savory
teriyaki flavors makes for a winning stir-fry.

⅓ cup soy sauce

2 tablespoons mirin

1 tablespoon minced ginger

1 tablespoon minced garlic

¼ cup chopped scallion

2 tablespoons vegetable oil,
preferably peanut

1 pound tempeh

1½ pounds bok choy,
chopped

½ cup vegetable stock (see
page 246) or water

¼ teaspoon salt

½ teaspoon pepper

1   Combine the soy sauce and mirin in a small saucepan with ⅓ cup
water. (If you don't have mirin, use maple syrup or other sweetener
and increase the water to ½ cup.) Cook over medium-low heat until
bubbling, about 2 minutes. Turn off the heat; stir in the ginger, garlic,
and scallion; and let sit.

2   Put the oil in a large skillet over medium-high heat. When it's hot,
crumble the tempeh into the pan and cook, stirring frequently and
breaking up the pieces, until they're browned, 5 to 7 minutes. Remove
the tempeh from the pan with a slotted spoon.

3   Return the skillet to the heat, add the bok choy, and cook, stirring
constantly, until it browns in places, 1 or 2 minutes. Add the stock.
Cook, stirring occasionally, until the bok choy is quite tender, 5 to
10 minutes, adding a bit more liquid only if necessary to keep the
vegetable from sticking.

4   Stir in 2 tablespoons of the teriyaki sauce and the tempeh and cook
until heated through, just 1 or 2 minutes. Taste and add the salt and
pepper (or more) if necessary and serve with remaining teriyaki sauce
on the side.

VARIATION

TERIYAKI BOK CHOY WITH EDAMAME Use 1½ cups frozen or fresh
edamame instead of tempeh.

MORE IDEAS

Any Asian greens work great in place of the bok choy: tatsoi, pea shoots,
Chinese broccoli, mizuna. (Red or green cabbage is also great in a pinch.)
• Up the *umami* factor by adding ½ pound sliced shiitake mushroom caps to
the tempeh after it starts to brown in Step 2. Stir-fry until they soften a bit,
another 1 or 2 minutes.

VEGETABLE POT PIE

MAKES 4 servings   **TIME** About 40 minutes

The tomato-based filling in the VB6 take on pot pie is loaded with vegetables and topped with phyllo for some crunch. Improvise as you like, using whatever veggies you've got in the fridge or freezer. Baking it in a square pan makes for easy prep and serving, but you could certainly divide the recipe among four 2-cup individual baking dishes for a more elegant presentation.

3 tablespoons olive oil

1 onion, chopped

2 carrots, chopped

1 red bell pepper, chopped

1 tablespoon minced garlic

½ teaspoon salt

¼ teaspoon pepper

One 15-ounce can diced tomatoes, drained (liquid reserved for another use)

½ pound green beans, chopped

1 pound chopped spinach

1½ cup peas (frozen are fine; don't bother to thaw)

1 tablespoon chopped fresh oregano, or 1 teaspoon dried

2 sheets whole wheat phyllo dough, thawed

1   Heat the oven to 375°F and grease a 2-quart or 9-inch-square baking pan with 1 tablespoon oil. Put another tablespoon of oil in a large pot over medium heat. Add the onion, carrots, and bell pepper, and cook, stirring occasionally, until they soften, 3 to 5 minutes.

2   Add the garlic, sprinkle with the salt and pepper, and cook, stirring until fragrant, no more than 1 minute. Add the tomatoes, bring to a boil, then stir in the beans and half of the spinach. Cook and stir just long enough for the spinach to soften and release its liquid, 1 or 2 minutes, then add the remaining spinach. When all the spinach is wilted, stir in the peas and then taste and adjust the seasoning and transfer the vegetables to the prepared pan. (You can cover and refrigerate the filling for up to a day; bring to room temperature before proceeding.)

3   Spread a sheet of phyllo on a cutting board and brush with 1 teaspoon oil; top with the second sheet and brush with another teaspoon oil. Fold the two phyllo sheets like a book, trim the sides to roughly fit your dish, and put over the vegetables. Score the top to let out steam. Brush the top with the remaining teaspoon oil.

4   Transfer the pot pie to the oven and bake until the crust is deeply golden and the filling is bubbling, 20 to 30 minutes. Serve hot or at room temperature.

VARIATIONS

VEGETABLE POT PIE WITH MASHED SWEET POTATO TOPPING
Instead of the phyllo sheets, roast or microwave 2 large sweet potatoes until very soft. Peel and mash them with the remaining tablespoon olive oil in Step 3 and a little more salt and pepper if you like. Use this mixture to top the filling, spreading to cover. Bake as directed.

AUTUMN VEGETABLE POT PIE   Omit the green beans. Swap 4 cups cubed pumpkin or butternut squash for the carrots, kale for the spinach, and corn for the peas.

EGGPLANT MEATBALLS

MAKES 4 servings   **TIME** About 1 hour, largely unattended

The more I play around with vegetable-based meatballs, the more I like
them; certainly they're not the same as meat meatballs, but the different
textures and flavors are terrific. To round out the meal for lunch, serve
these over pasta, rice, salad, or steamed greens with a squeeze of lemon.

3 tablespoons olive oil

1 pound eggplant,
unpeeled, cut into cubes no
larger than 1 inch

1 teaspoon salt

½ teaspoon pepper

1 onion, chopped

1 tablespoon minced garlic

1 cup cooked or canned
white beans (see page 232)

¼ cup chopped fresh
parsley

1 cup breadcrumbs,
preferably whole wheat
(see page 251)

Pinch red chile flakes
(optional)

2 cups All-Purpose Tomato
Sauce (page 238)

1   Heat the oven to 375°F. Use 1 tablespoon olive oil to grease a
large rimmed baking sheet. Put 1 tablespoon oil in a large skillet over
medium-high heat. When it's hot, add the eggplant and ¼ cup water.
Sprinkle with the salt and pepper and cook, stirring occasionally, until
the pieces shrivel a bit and are tender and beginning to color, 10 to
15 minutes. Transfer the eggplant to the bowl of a food processor.

2   Add the remaining 1 tablespoon oil to the pan along with the onion
and garlic and return to the heat. Cook, stirring frequently, until they're
soft and translucent, 3 to 5 minutes. Meanwhile, drain the beans; if
using canned, rinse them before draining. Add the beans and parsley
to the work bowl with the eggplant and pulse until well combined and
chopped, but not pureed.

3   Toss the eggplant mixture with the onion and garlic, then add the
breadcrumbs and red chile flakes if you're using them. Taste and adjust
the seasoning. Roll the mixture into 12 balls about 2 inches in diameter;
transfer them to the prepared pan. Bake, undisturbed, until they're firm
and well browned, 25 to 30 minutes.

4   Meanwhile, warm the tomato sauce. Serve the meatballs hot or at
room temperature along with the tomato sauce.

VARIATIONS

MUSHROOM MEATBALLS For those who don't fancy eggplant, or just
as a change, substitute 1 pound chopped mushrooms of any kind for the
eggplant. In Step 1, cook them until the pan is dry and they start to stick
a bit, 5 to 10 minutes. Then mix, form, and bake as in the original recipe.

CAULIFLOWER MEATBALLS Substitute 1 pound chopped cauliflower
for the eggplant; core and roughly chop it. In Step 1, cook the pieces
until the pan is dry and they start to brown a bit, 10 to 15 minutes. Then
mix, form, and bake as in the original recipe.

MORE IDEAS

The coarser the breadcrumbs are, the better. If you can't make your own, use
panko (preferably whole wheat if you can find it).

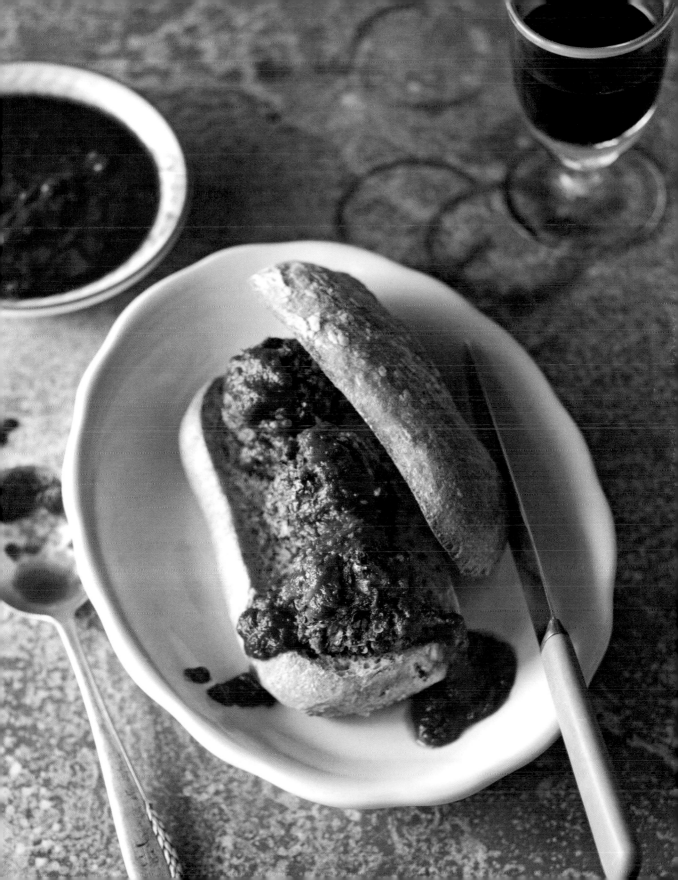

P.L.T. SANDWICH

MAKES **4 servings**   TIME **45 minutes**

Portabello. Lettuce. Tomato. The mushroom "bacon" is chewy, meaty (it's
a cliché to say that about mushrooms, but it's true), and so easy to make;
you'll want to double the batch and keep it handy in the fridge for topping
salads and rice or noodle bowls, scrambling with tofu for breakfast, or
adding to beans and vegetable stews. But start with this sandwich.

2 tablespoons olive oil

1½ pounds whole
portabello mushrooms

1 teaspoon smoked paprika

¾ teaspoon salt

½ teaspoon pepper

8 slices whole wheat bread,
toasted

¼ cup Vegannaise
(page 242)

16 (or so) iceberg or
romaine lettuce leaves

2 large tomatoes, sliced
crosswise

1 Heat the oven to 400°F and position two racks so there's at least a
few inches in between them. Line two rimmed baking sheets with foil
and smear each with 1 tablespoon olive oil. Remove the stems from the
mushrooms and save them for another use. Slice the caps crosswise as
thin as you can manage; transfer them to the prepared sheets.

2 Spread out the mushrooms into a single layer and sprinkle with
the paprika, salt, and pepper. Transfer the pans to the oven and roast,
undisturbed, until the mushrooms release their water and the pan is
almost dry again, 20 to 30 minutes.

3 Lower the heat to 325°F and continue to cook the slices undisturbed
until they dry and shrivel a bit, and release evenly from the pan, another
5 to 10 minutes. Let the mushrooms cool to room temperature or eat
them hot. To assemble the sandwiches, spread both pieces of the bread
with Vegannaise, put lettuce on one slice and tomato and mushroom
slices on the other; close, cut in half if you like, and serve.

VARIATIONS

E.L.T. SANDWICH Eggplant bacon takes a little longer to prepare but is
really great. Again, you will find plenty of uses for leftovers: Use closer
to 2 pounds; don't bother to peel. Halve, cut crosswise into thin slices,
and season and roast as described for the mushrooms.

OPEN-FACE P.L.T. OR E.L.T. SANDWICH Up the salad factor—start
with one slice of toasted bread, followed by the mushrooms. Top with
2 cups salad greens, the tomato slice, and any cooked or raw chopped
vegetables you like. Dress with the dollop of Vegannaise and a squeeze
of lemon or splash of wine vinegar.

MORE IDEAS

Try other mushrooms: If you can find king oyster or pom-pom mushrooms,
grab 'em. Oyster and shiitake mushrooms make good "bacon bits." • Add
garnishes: Layer on thinly sliced pickled vegetables or onion, grated carrots,
or chopped radishes. • Change the condiment: Use mustard, miso, Sriracha,
or pureed herbs instead of the Vegannaise.

PHONY BOLOGNA

MAKES 8 servings   **TIME** A little more than 2½ hours, almost entirely unattended, plus time for chilling

Vegan processed food is still junk in my book, which is why I can't advocate for those deli-meat substitutes. (Have you read the labels?) But I recognize the importance of being able to eat a sandwich. So instead I suggest you take 10 minutes to whip up this homemade tofu loaf, and then spend the baking time doing something else. The results are shockingly like bologna—only square!—especially if you fry the slices in a little olive oil. You'll have enough for a week's worth of brown bagging.

1 tablespoon vegetable oil

2 pounds firm tofu
(2 blocks), cut into chunks

12 ounces silken tofu
(¾ cup)

¼ cup tomato paste

1 tablespoon maple syrup

1 teaspoon garlic powder

2 tablespoons smoked paprika

1 teaspoon salt

½ teaspoon pepper

¼ teaspoon allspice

1 Heat the oven to 300°F. Grease a 9 by 5-inch loaf pan with the oil. Put all the remaining ingredients in a food processor and let the machine run for 1 minute. Stop to scrape down the sides of the work bowl and repeat once or twice more, until the mixture is completely smooth and evenly colored.

2 Spoon the tofu mixture into the prepared pan, spreading and pressing to eliminate air pockets; smooth the top as best as you can.

3 Put the pan on a rimmed baking sheet and transfer to the oven. Bake the bologna until the sides brown and separate from the pan and the top puffs and forms a crust (don't worry if it cracks a bit), about 2½ hours. Let cool completely before inverting from the pan; for the best results refrigerate for several hours before slicing. (The bologna will keep in the fridge for about a week, or in the freezer for months; if you're storing some, wait to slice it until just before using.)

VARIATION

PHONY MORTADELLA You'll be amazed. Hold back ½ tofu brick, then cut and puree the rest. Cut the reserved piece into ½-inch cubes. After pureeing the tofu and spices in Step 1, fold in the cubed tofu and ¼ cup chopped pistachios. Shape and bake as for the original recipe.

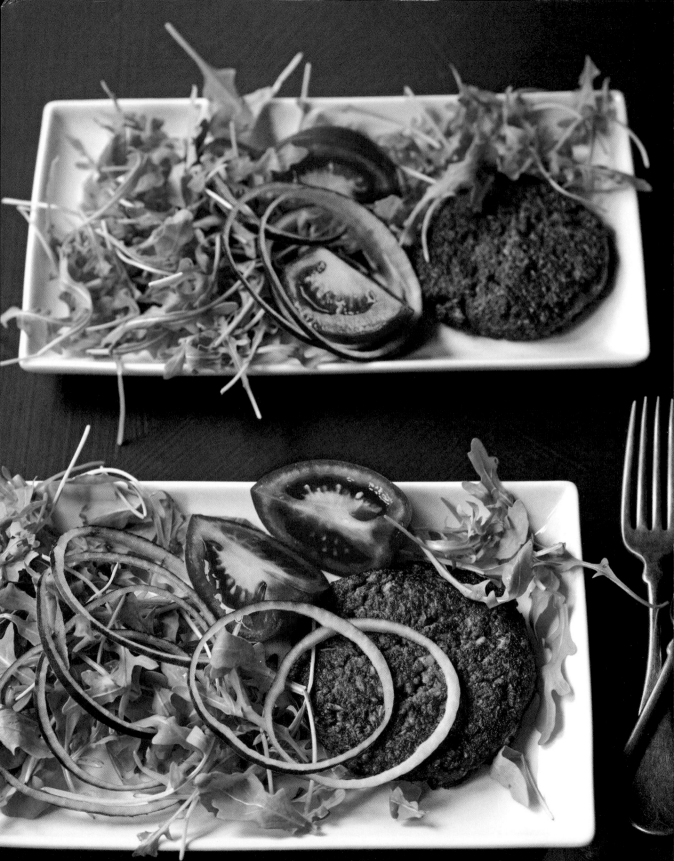

MUSHROOM-NUT BURGERS OVER GREENS

MAKES 4 servings   **TIME** 30 minutes

I've made tons of meatless burgers since becoming a part-time vegan, and they're always better than store-bought. Almost as convenient too: Just double or triple the batch and freeze the burgers on a wax paper–lined tray until solid; then wrap them up and keep them frozen for a rainy day. You could also have them on a whole-grain bun.

1 cup rolled oats (not quick-cooking or instant)

2 (or more) garlic cloves

1 pound mushrooms (like cremini or button), trimmed and halved

½ cup pecans (or any other nut you like)

2 teaspoons chili powder

½ teaspoon salt

¼ teaspoon pepper

2 tablespoons vegetable oil

3 tablespoons fresh lemon juice

8 cups torn lettuce or other salad greens

2 tomatoes, cut into wedges

½ large red onion, sliced into thin rings

1 Put the oats in a food processor and let the machine run until they're ground to a coarse meal, about 1 minute. Transfer them to a large bowl.

2 Pulse the garlic in the food processor (no need to wash it first) until the cloves are broken up a bit, then add the mushrooms. Pulse until the mixture is finely chopped but not pureed. Add the mushrooms and garlic to the bowl with the oats. Put the nuts in the food processor (again, no need to wash it) and let the machine run until they're ground to a thick paste, adding water a teaspoon at a time if necessary just to let the machine do its job; be careful not to make the mixture too wet. Scrape the nut butter into the bowl with a rubber spatula.

3 Add the chili powder, salt, and pepper and stir with the spatula, pressing and folding as you work until the ingredients are distributed evenly. Refrigerate the mixture for 10 minutes, then make four patties.

4 Put the oil in a large skillet (preferably nonstick or cast-iron) over medium heat. When it's hot, add the burgers and cook, undisturbed, until they're browned on the bottom and release evenly from the pan, 3 to 5 minutes. Turn the burgers, lower the heat a bit, and cook on the other side until firm and browned, 3 to 5 minutes more.

5 Remove the burgers and return the pan to the heat with the lemon juice and ½ cup water. Cook, stirring constantly, until the liquid thickens a bit. Serve the burgers on a bed of lettuce, drizzled with the pan sauce and topped with the tomatoes and onions.

VARIATIONS

MISO-MUSHROOM BURGERS Instead of the nuts, grind together ¼ cup chopped walnuts and ¼ cup any miso. Use several fresh ginger slices instead of the garlic and add 1 or more tablespoons soy sauce to the pan sauce with the lemon juice in Step 5.

TAHINI-MUSHROOM BURGERS Use tahini instead of the nuts and add it to the mixture in Step 3. Substitute cumin for the chili powder.

SNACKS

GORPCORN

WASABIMAME

COCKTAIL CHICKPEAS

MANCHURIAN TORTILLA CRISPS

KOREAN-STYLE CUCUMBER
QUICKLES

ENDIVE WITH MUSHROOM-OLIVE
TAPENADE

CUCUMBERS WITH CARROT-
GINGER-MISO DIP

CARROTS WITH CHIPOTLE "MAYO"

SOUTHWESTERN BEAN DIP WITH
PEPPERS

RADISHES WITH AVOCADO DIP

TOFU JERKY, THE SEQUEL

FRUIT CANDY

FROZEN TROPICAL TRUFFLES

RASPBERRY SORBET ON A STICK

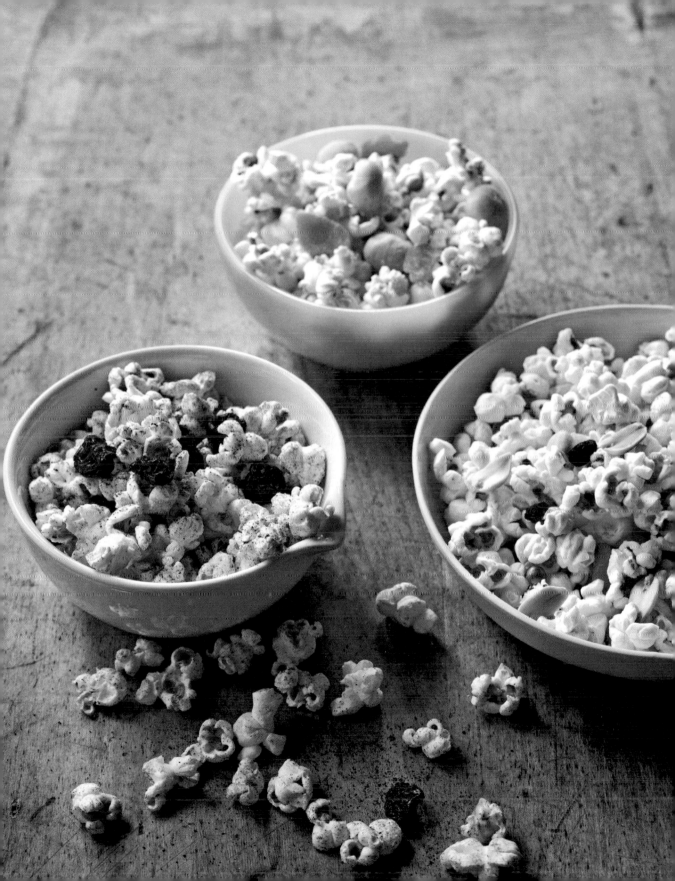

There's absolutely nothing wrong with snacking—as long as you're reaching for Unlimited Foods like fruits and vegetables augmented with small amounts of flexible foods like whole grains, beans, or nuts. It could well be that once you start eating better your between-meal cravings will change dramatically and avoiding junk foods won't be a big deal. I definitely found that to be the case. Nevertheless, here are a few tips to help you avoid pitfalls. They may sound like common sense, but they're worth repeating because they really work.

First and foremost: Keep a few pieces of washed fruit on the counter or at your desk at work. And if you have the discipline to cut up and portion fruit to store in the fridge so it's ready to eat, all the better. Make sure there's frozen fruit handy too; you can use it right from the freezer.

Likewise with vegetables: Trim, rinse, peel, and cut up whatever you need so all you have to do is open the fridge. Keep carrots, radishes, and celery in a bowl of water; store the rest in airtight containers. (For dips, see the string of recipes starting on page 140.)

In the Flexible Foods category, I reach for nuts. Not over and over again, mind you, but a handful. Portion them out ahead of time if you think limiting your intake is going to be an issue. You can also keep crisp roasted beans at home or at work. (There are two recipes on pages 135 and 136 so you don't have to rely on store-bought.) And by all means use the microwave: With a VB6 mindset, cooked vegetables drizzled with a little olive oil and sprinkled with salt make satisfying snacks, as do last night's leftover side dishes.

And finally, try the recipes in this chapter. All can be made ahead of time, stored, and easily transported.

GORPCORN

MAKES 4 servings   TIME 10 minutes

A combination of two of my favorite treats: popcorn and gorp. Simple whole grains, legumes, and fruits, tossed together to become a nutritious, addictive, and practically guilt-free snack.

2 tablespoons vegetable oil

½ cup popping corn

1 cup raisins

1 teaspoon salt

1 cup raw unsalted peanuts

1 Put the oil in a large pot and turn the heat to medium; add 3 corn kernels and cover.

2 When the kernels pop, remove the lid and add the remaining popcorn. Cover and slide the pot back and forth over the burner, holding the lid in place until the corn begins to pop. Cook, continuing to shake the pot occasionally, until the popping sound stops, 3 to 5 minutes. Transfer the popcorn to a large bowl, add the raisins, sprinkle with the salt, and toss.

3 Put the pot back on the stove over medium-low heat. Add the nuts and cook, shaking the pan until they're fragrant and just beginning to brown, 1 or 2 minutes. Add the nuts to the bowl with the popcorn and raisins and toss again. Serve immediately (or store in an airtight container for up to a couple of days).

VARIATIONS

MICROWAVE GORPCORN Cut the ingredients in half and figure two servings instead of four. Use roasted peanuts if you want to save an additional step. Combine ¼ cup popping corn with ¼ teaspoon salt in a medium microwave-safe dish or popcorn popper designed for the microwave. Microwave on high for 2 to 3 minutes, until there are 4 or 5 seconds between pops. Open the dish container carefully because steam will have built up. While the popcorn is warm, transfer it to a bowl and toss with ½ cup each peanuts and raisins and ½ teaspoon salt.

CHILE-CHERRY GORPCORN In Step 2, when you add the salt, sprinkle the popcorn with 1 tablespoon chili powder (with or without a pinch of ground red chile or cayenne), and toss with dried cherries instead of the raisins.

KETTLE GORPCORN Especially good with hazelnuts or pecans instead of peanuts. In Step 2, before transferring the popcorn to the bowl, drizzle it with 2 tablespoons maple syrup and toss it in the pot. Add 1 teaspoon cinnamon along with the salt.

(recipe continues)

BASIL GORPCORN Try this with cashews instead of peanuts and use unsweetened coconut (ribbons are better than flakes) instead of raisins. In Step 2, before transferring the popcorn to the bowl, toss it with ½ cup chopped fresh basil.

MEDITERRANEAN GORPCORN Use olive oil instead of vegetable oil to pop the corn and substitute almonds for the peanuts and chopped apricots or dates (or a combination) for the raisins. Add 1 teaspoon cumin along with the salt in Step 2.

SEAWEED GORPCORN Walnuts are a good substitute for the peanuts here. In Step 3, when the nuts are just about toasted, add ½ cup shredded nori, arame, or dulse to the pot to cook for the last 30 seconds or so.

TROPICAL GORPCORN Substitute macadamia nuts for the peanuts and chopped dried mango, pineapple, or papaya for the raisins. Add ¼ cup unsweetened coconut ribbons along with the fruit in Step 2.

WASABIMAME

MAKES **4 servings**   TIME **30 minutes**

No doubt you've eaten those spicy fried peas coated with wasabi. These roasted edamame snacks are a lot like those, only heartier and with a more interesting texture. They are not only a satisfying snack (they're loaded with protein) but also make a fine garnish for salads, soups, and rice or noodle bowls.

3 cups shelled fresh or frozen edamame

2 tablespoons vegetable oil

2 teaspoons wasabi powder, or more to taste

1 teaspoon salt

1   Heat the oven to 400°F. Dry the edamame as well as possible, toss them with the oil, and spread them on a rimmed baking sheet.

2   Roast the beans, shaking the pan to roll them around once or twice, until they're colored and crisp, 25 to 30 minutes. Sprinkle with the wasabi and salt and toss with a spatula until they're evenly coated. Return the pan to the oven until the wasabi toasts a bit and becomes fragrant, another 3 to 5 minutes. Let cool completely, shaking the pan occasionally; they'll crisp even more. Serve right away (or store in an airtight container for up to 1 week).

VARIATIONS

MUSTARDAMAME If you don't like wasabi or find it too overwhelming, try using powdered mustard instead.

SRIRACHAMAME Substitute 1 tablespoon of sriracha for the wasabi powder.

WASABI PEAS Use fresh or frozen peas instead of edamame.

SOY EDAMAME Omit the salt. Once the beans have cooled and crisped, drizzle them with 2 tablespoons soy sauce and toss to coat.

MORE IDEAS

Olive or sesame oil can be good substitutes for the vegetable oil, depending what other flavorings you choose. • Other seasonings to try instead of wasabi powder: black pepper, garlic powder, red chile flakes (or ground red chile), spice blends like curry, five-spice, or chili powder, and grated citrus zest.
• Swap out sesame seeds or finely chopped nuts for the wasabi powder or other seasonings.

COCKTAIL CHICKPEAS

MAKES 4 servings   **TIME** 25 minutes

The spicy curry-based coating makes these nutlike tidbits a natural for snacking. But you don't have to have an adult beverage in your hand to enjoy them. They're great as a garnish for salads and soups too, or any time in the afternoon.

As always, home-cooked chickpeas will have the best flavor and texture, but you can use canned with good results. Either way, be sure to drain the chickpeas as thoroughly as possible and dry them gently with a clean towel before roasting them or they won't get crisp.

3 cups cooked or canned chickpeas

2 tablespoons olive oil

1 tablespoon curry powder

½ teaspoon salt

¼ teaspoon pepper

1   Heat the oven to 450°F. Drain the chickpeas; if canned, rinse them before draining. Dry the chickpeas well, then put them on a rimmed baking sheet and transfer to the oven. Cook, shaking the pan as necessary, until the beans begin to brown evenly, 15 to 25 minutes. The browner they get, the crisper they'll be.

2   When the chickpeas are as dark as you want them, drizzle them with the olive oil; sprinkle with the curry, salt, and pepper; and toss with a spatula until they're well coated. Return them to the oven and turn off the heat. Let them sit until the curry powder is fragrant but not burned, no more than 3 minutes. Remove the pan; the chickpeas will crisp as they sit. Serve right away (or store in an airtight container in the fridge for up to 1 week).

VARIATION

SALT AND VINEGAR CHICKPEAS Start by putting the chickpeas in a medium saucepan with 1 cup cider vinegar and 2 cups water; bring to a boil, then cover the pot and let the beans sit for at least 5 and up to 15 minutes. Then drain and dry the beans and proceed with the recipe from Step 1, omitting the curry powder.

MORE IDEAS

Try other spice blends or individual spices instead of the curry: five-spice, chili powder, garam masala, or garlic powder. • Instead of chickpeas, use cannellini or big white limas or other oversized beans.

MANCHURIAN TORTILLA CRISPS

MAKES 4 servings   TIME About 30 minutes

A couple of twists on the wildly popular tomato-y tortilla chips from *VB6*.
Here I've played with Asian flavors in the main recipes, but be sure to
check out the alternatives below too. The combinations are as crazy as the
stuff you buy in a bag, but these are based on real food and are fresh as
they can be.

¼ cup tomato paste

2 tablespoons sesame oil

1 teaspoon soy sauce

¼ teaspoon pepper

Eight 6-inch corn tortillas

1   Heat the oven to 350°F. Combine the tomato paste, sesame oil, soy
sauce, and pepper in a small bowl. Put the tortillas on a baking sheet
(or two) and use your fingers or a brush to smear a thin layer of the
tomato mixture onto the top of each.

2   Bake until the tortillas are as chewy or crisp as you like them and
the tops have darkened slightly, 20 to 25 minutes. Break the tortillas
into pieces if you like. Serve warm (or store in an airtight container at
room temperature for up to a few days).

VARIATIONS

LIME TORTILLA CRISPS Omit the tomato paste, sesame oil, and soy
sauce. Instead combine 1 tablespoon grated lime zest (from about
2 limes), 2 tablespoons olive oil, ½ teaspoon salt, and ¼ teaspoon
pepper and use that to dress the tortillas before baking. Reduce the
baking time to 15 to 20 minutes.

GARLIC TORTILLAS Omit the tomato paste, sesame oil, and soy sauce.
Bake the tortillas with 2 tablespoons olive oil, ½ teaspoon salt, and
¼ teaspoon pepper. Reduce the baking time to 15 to 20 minutes. Once
they're out of the oven, rub the tortillas with the cut surfaces of halved
raw garlic cloves.

KOREAN-STYLE CUCUMBER QUICKLES

MAKES 2 cups pickles   TIME 45 minutes, plus time for chilling

Here, two crazes—canning and Korean food—collide. The result is an easily made pickle that requires neither fancy equipment nor weird ingredients. The balance of sweet and salty makes this a perfectly satisfying snack
or a tantalizing appetizer. For the best results, please plan ahead: These
pickles are technically ready to eat in about 45 minutes, but they benefit
greatly from marinating for at least several hours in the refrigerator.

1½ pounds cucumbers

1 tablespoon sesame seeds

½ cup apple cider vinegar

2 tablespoons minced garlic

2 tablespoons maple syrup
or other sweetener

1 teaspoon red chile flakes,
or more to taste

1½ teaspoons salt

1   Peel the cucumbers if the skins are thick or waxed, and cut them
into 2- or 3-inch spears or crosswise into rounds about ½ inch thick.

2   Put the sesame seeds in a large nonreactive pot over medium-high
heat. Cook, shaking the pot nearly constantly, until they're fragrant and
begin to darken a little, 1 or 2 minutes. Remove them from the pot.

3   Add the vinegar, garlic, syrup, red chile flakes, and salt to the pot
along with 2 cups water, and bring to a boil. Put the cucumbers and
sesame seeds in the pot and remove from the heat. Let the vegetables
sit in the brine for 30 minutes, stirring once or twice to make sure
they're all covered at least part of the time. Transfer to jars or other
airtight containers and refrigerate for up to a week.

VARIATIONS

GIARDINERA   The Italian classic made simple. Use peppercorns
instead of the sesame seeds, red wine vinegar instead of the cider
vinegar, and add 1 tablespoon chopped fresh oregano or rosemary in
Step 3. Decrease the salt to 1 teaspoon. Try pickling cauliflower, fennel,
carrots, or bell peppers—alone or in combination—in Step 3 instead of
the cucumbers if you like.

JAPANESE-STYLE MUSHROOM QUICKLES   Substitute halved
mushrooms for the cucumbers and ginger for the garlic. Use rice
vinegar instead of cider vinegar; increase the vinegar to ¾ cup and
reduce the water to 1¾ cups. In Step 3, after you remove the pot from
the heat, stir in 2 tablespoons any miso paste.

FRENCH-STYLE RADISH QUICKLES   Use halved radishes instead
of the cucumbers, white wine vinegar instead of the cider vinegar,
and 1 chopped shallot or scallion in place of the sesame seeds; add
2 tablespoons chopped fresh tarragon. Skip the maple syrup and red
chile flakes and increase the salt to 1 teaspoon.

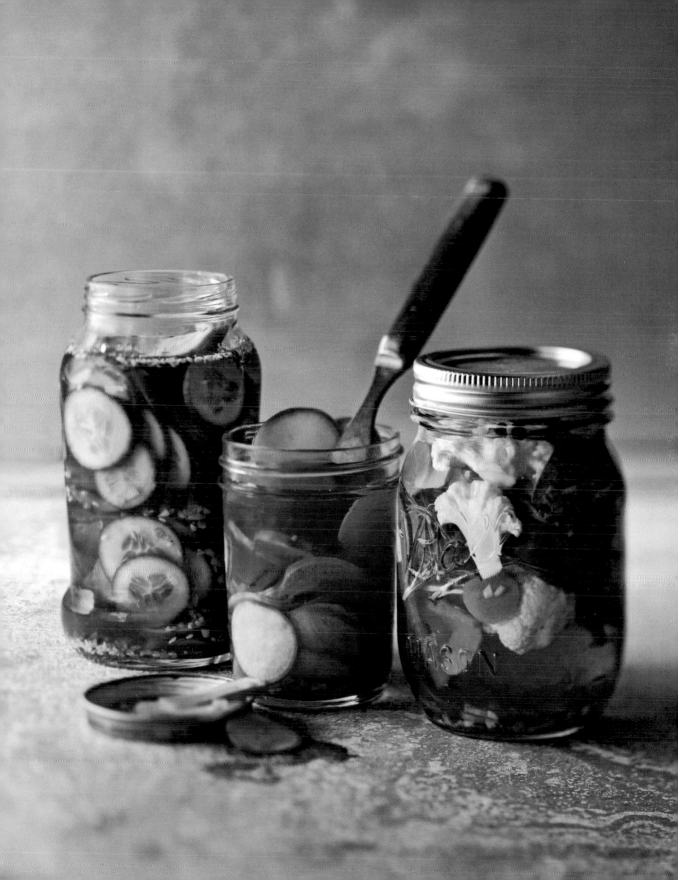

ENDIVE WITH MUSHROOM-OLIVE TAPENADE

MAKES 4 servings   TIME 20 minutes

Here's a great dip-and-chip combo. The dip is briny and savory with a hearty texture not unlike pâté. Pair it with crisp, subtle endive leaves for an elegant and effortless combination. It's also terrific on thin slices of whole wheat toast or as a garnish for cooked vegetables.

1 pound endive

4 ounces black olives, preferably oil-cured, pitted

1 pound fresh mushrooms (like cremini or button), halved

2 tablespoons capers, rinsed and drained if salted, drained if brined

1 (or more) garlic clove, smashed

3 tablespoons olive oil

½ teaspoon pepper

½ cup chopped fresh parsley (optional)

1   Trim the bottom of each endive so you can separate the leaves. Rinse the leaves in cold water and drain in a colander or on towels until they're as dry as possible.

2   Put all the remaining ingredients (including the parsley if you're using it) in a food processor. Pulse the machine until you get a rough puree with bits of mushrooms and olives still visible. To serve, put a small bowl of the tapenade on a platter with the endive around it for dipping. (Or pack everything away in the fridge and eat it as an afternoon snack.)

VARIATIONS

MUSHROOM-GREEN OLIVE TAPENADE   Substitute green olives for black. Add 1 teaspoon ground cumin and the grated zest of ½ lemon.

MUSHROOM-DRIED TOMATO TAPENADE   Replace the olives with roughly chopped dried tomatoes (see page 229) or store-bought dried tomatoes. Use 1 cup fresh basil leaves instead of the parsley.

MORE IDEAS

Other vegetables are also fine vehicles for getting the dip to your mouth: Try sliced fennel, carrot coins, celery sticks, or thin slices of jícama. • Add nuts: ½ cup toasted pine nuts, walnuts, or almonds are a great addition for some crunchy texture. • Add another layer of flavor with another herb—like fresh thyme, rosemary, sage, or oregano—either in addition to or instead of the parsley. Figure no more than 1 tablespoon chopped fresh herbs.

CUCUMBERS WITH CARROT-GINGER-MISO DIP

MAKES 4 servings   TIME 15 minutes

Umami, the "fifth taste," is a savory quality that registers on your palate much the same way as do sweet, salty, sour, and bitter flavors. You find it in meat, mushrooms, soy sauce—and, for sure, miso. This dip packs a load of *umami*, balanced with the tang of rice vinegar and the sweetness of carrots—a wonderful foil for cool cucumbers. It is also a fantastic marinade or glaze for grilled vegetables, tofu, chicken, or meat.

1½ pounds cucumbers

1 large carrot, cut into chunks

1 inch ginger, peeled

2 tablespoons any miso, plus more to taste

½ cup warm water

¼ cup rice vinegar

1 tablespoon mirin

½ teaspoon pepper

1 Peel the cucumbers if their skins are thick or waxed and cut them crosswise on the bias into coins about ½ inch thick. Refrigerate them while you make the dip.

2 Put the carrots in a food processor and pulse a few times to mince. Add the remaining ingredients and let the machine run for a minute or so until the mixture is relatively smooth. Taste and add more miso if you'd like and pulse again. Serve immediately with the cucumbers. (Or store the components in airtight containers and refrigerate for up to 1 day.)

VARIATIONS

MISO-CARROT HERB DIPPING SAUCE Substitute ½ cup minced fresh cilantro, basil, Thai basil, or mint (or a combination) for the ginger.

MISO-CARROT CITRUS DIPPING SAUCE Instead of the rice vinegar, use fresh lemon, lime, orange, or tangerine juice. If you like, grate some of the zest and float a sprinkle on top of the dip.

MISO-CARROT SOY DIPPING SAUCE Want something a little saltier? Add a tablespoon or 2 of soy sauce.

MISO-CARROT VINAIGRETTE Transform this into a bona fide salad dressing by adding 4 teaspoons peanut oil and 2 teaspoons sesame oil to the food processor with the vinegar in Step 2.

MORE IDEAS

Other vegetables to try with this dip: daikon or other radishes, celery, or raw or parboiled cauliflower or broccoli florets.

CARROTS WITH CHIPOTLE "MAYO"

MAKES 4 servings **TIME** 10 minutes

Talk about a stellar dip. The first time I made this it sparked a debate about whether it was "real" mayonnaise. But vegan "mayo"—or vegan-naise, as it's usually called—is a creamy, vibrant staple you will want to have on hand to spruce up vegetables, use as a springboard for a creamy salad dressing, or spread on a sandwich. There's a basic recipe on page 242, but here I spin that formula into a spicy and colorful complement for sweet, crunchy carrots.

8 ounces silken tofu (about 1 cup)

2 tablespoons olive oil

¼ cup fresh lime juice

½ teaspoon salt

1 canned chipotle chile and some of the adobo sauce, plus more to taste

1 pound carrots, cut into coins or sticks

1 Put all the ingredients except the carrots in a blender. Puree, stopping once or twice to scrape down the sides of the container with a rubber spatula, until the tofu is completely smooth and evenly colored. This could take several minutes and you may need to add 1 or 2 table-spoons of water to help the machine do its work.

2 When the mixture is ready, taste and adjust the seasoning. For a little more heat, add another chipotle or more of the adobo sauce and blend again. Serve right away or refrigerate the dip and carrots separately (they'll keep up to a couple days).

VARIATIONS

JÍCAMA WITH JALAPEÑO "MAYO" Skip the chipotle and add 2 seeded fresh jalapeño chiles to the blender in Step 1. Peel a 1-pound jícama and cut it into sticks to use for dipping.

DAIKON WITH MISO "MAYO" Use 3 tablespoons miso paste (or more to taste) instead of the chipotle and lemon juice instead of the lime juice. Substitute daikon for the carrots; cut them into coins or sticks.

MAKING CRUDITÉS MORE CONVENIENT

A fridge full of ready-to-eat vegetables—calling them crudités elevates their stature—is a lot more exciting than carrot and celery sticks. Anything from the plant world that you cut up and pop in your mouth, whether you dip it, stir-fry it, or toss it into a salad, qualifies as crudités in my book.

It's easy to keep prepared vegetables fresh. Use a bowl of water for sliced carrots, celery, radishes, fennel, or kohlrabi (surprisingly good raw). After you cut up cucumbers, bell pepper, or zucchini and other summer squash, put them in a sealed container in the crisper.

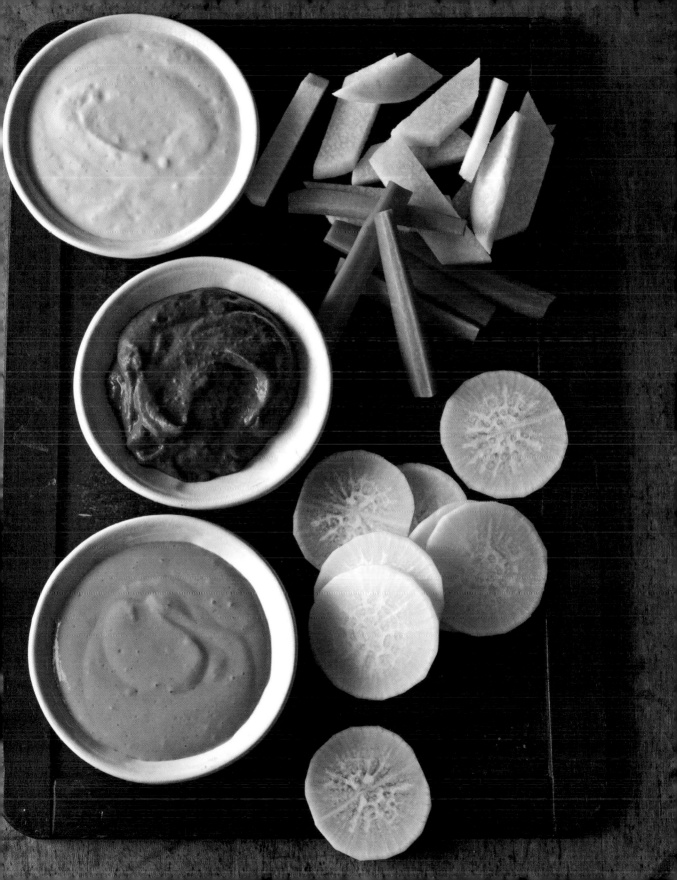

SOUTHWESTERN BEAN DIP WITH PEPPERS

MAKES 4 servings   TIME 10 minutes with cooked or canned beans

Commercial bean dips generally aren't too bad, but when you make them yourself with fresh, real ingredients, they become healthy vegan snacks that are still loads of fun. If you've never made one from scratch, you're going to be amazed with the difference in flavor and the range of possible textures. All of these (see the variations) are terrific.

3 cups cooked or canned black beans (see page 232)

1 small white onion, quartered

1 garlic clove, smashed

1 cup packed cilantro sprigs

2 tablespoons fresh lime juice

2 teaspoons chili powder

½ teaspoon salt

¼ teaspoon pepper

1 pound bell peppers, any color, cut into sticks

1   Drain the beans. If you made them yourself, reserve the cooking liquid; if they're canned, discard it and rinse the beans. Put all the ingredients except the peppers in a blender or food processor and puree, adding water (or the reserved bean cooking liquid if you've got some) as needed to make a smooth but not watery dip. (If you want a lumpier texture, mash the beans in a bowl with a fork or potato masher, then mince and add the remaining ingredients and stir together by hand.)

2   Taste and adjust the seasoning if necessary. Serve the dip at room temperature, refrigerate it until cold, or warm it in a small pot over medium-low heat (or in the microwave oven). Serve with the bell pepper sticks for dipping.

VARIATIONS

ROSEMARY-WHITE BEAN DIP WITH FENNEL   Use white beans instead of black, skip the onion, and increase the garlic to 2 cloves. Substitute the leaves from 1 sprig fresh rosemary leaves for the cilantro, and lemon juice for the lime juice. Omit the chili powder. Serve the dip with fennel sticks.

CHIPOTLE-PINTO BEAN DIP WITH JÍCAMA   Use pinto, not black, beans. Omit the onion. Instead of the chili powder use 1 (or more) canned chipotle chile with some of the accompanying adobo. Garnish the dip with chopped scallions and serve with jícama sticks.

SPANISH-STYLE CHICKPEA DIP WITH CARROTS   Use chickpeas instead of the black beans. Swap ½ cup fresh parsley for the cilantro, 1 tablespoon sherry vinegar for the lime juice, and smoked paprika for the chili powder. Garnish the dip with chopped almonds and serve with carrot sticks.

THREE WAYS TO PUREE

To transform something chunky—like soup or tender cooked vegetables or fruit—into something smooth, you need one of three machines: an immersion blender, a food processor, or a tabletop blender. Each has its pros and cons:

An immersion blender (an ultra-light handheld device that functions as an upside-down blender) is the least expensive and is perfect for working through a pot of soup, but not much more.

Upright blenders are much more versatile and high powered, capable of grinding ice and hard raw foods, as well as pulverizing bread and some grains.

The most versatile (and expensive) is the food processor, which can do everything from grate cheese and mince vegetables to knead dough and turn frozen fruit into sorbet. (These don't, however, hold much liquid and never really create as smooth a puree as you'll get with a blender.)

If you're going to make smoothies, where there's frozen fruit and ice involved, you've really got to use a blender. See the recipes starting on page 48. And for quick frozen treats like the recipes on pages 152 and 208, a food processor is the only way to go.

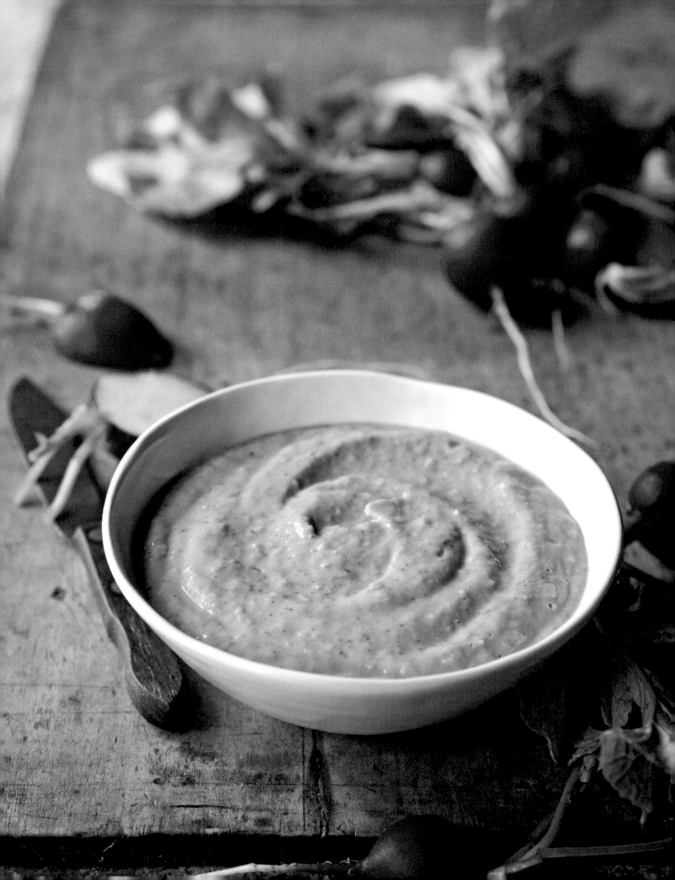

RADISHES WITH AVOCADO DIP

MAKES 4 servings   TIME 10 minutes, plus time to chill

With its surprising mash-up of flavors and textures, this dip combines perfectly with the sharp bite of radishes to wake up your taste buds. Ditto anything intensely flavored, like sliced poblano chiles, roasted sweet potato, or salted tortilla chips. If you want something a bit more mellow, pair this dip with wide matchsticks of jícama or carrots.

2 pounds radishes, preferably with greens attached

1 large avocado, halved and pitted

2 ounces silken tofu (¼ cup)

1 small bunch fresh cilantro, tender stems and leaves

1 garlic clove, smashed

1 tablespoon fresh lime juice

1 fresh hot chile (like jalapeño), seeded

5 or 6 tomatillos, husks removed

½ teaspoon salt

1   Scrub the radishes well and trim off the bottoms and greens, leaving about 1 inch of the stems attached if you're using whole radishes so there's something to hold when you dip. Put them in the fridge to chill.

2   Scoop the avocado flesh into a blender and add the tofu, cilantro, garlic, lime juice, chile, tomatillos, and salt in a blender; puree until smooth, stopping to scrape down the sides of the container as needed. Taste and adjust the seasoning.

3   To serve, transfer the mixture to a shallow bowl and serve with the radishes on the side.

VARIATIONS

CHARRED TOMATILLO DIP Before blending the ingredients, turn on the broiler and set the rack 4 inches from the heat source. Broil the tomatillos, garlic, and jalapeño for a few minutes, turning once, until charred. Remove the garlic as soon as it's toasted to avoid a bitter taste. Let the ingredients cool, then proceed with the recipe.

SPINACH-AVOCADO DIP Put 1 tablespoon olive oil in a skillet over medium-high heat. Add the garlic, minced instead, and 2 cups of spinach; sauté until wilted. Remove the spinach and garlic from the pan and let cool. Substitute lemon juice for the lime juice and skip the jalapeño and cilantro. Top with chopped tomatoes and scallions.

CURRIED MANGO DIP Use a mango instead of the avocado and add 2 teaspoons curry powder to the blender before pureeing. Serve with the radishes or with cucumber spears.

MORE IDEAS

Other options for dippers: carrot, celery, kohlrabi, or jícama sticks.

TOFU JERKY, THE SEQUEL

MAKES 4 servings   **TIME** About 1 hour, largely unattended

One of my favorite snacks from *VB6* is now an ongoing project, as I continue to play with jerky variations. It's a portable, chewy snack that's the next best thing—flavor, not healthwise!—to a Slim Jim. And it's easy to make, too.

1 pound firm tofu (1 block)

1 tablespoon tomato paste

1 teaspoon soy sauce

½ teaspoons cumin

½ teaspoon smoked paprika

2 teaspoons brown sugar

½ teaspoon salt

¼ teaspoon chili powder

1   Heat the oven to 225°F. Line a baking sheet with parchment paper or a silicon mat. Cut the block of tofu in half through the equator and blot the halves dry. Then cut each half the long way into slices a bit thicker than ⅛ inch (you should have about 28 slices total), and lay them on the parchment (it's preferable if they're touching).

2   Bake the tofu for 30 minutes. Meanwhile, stir together the remaining ingredients with 1 tablespoon water to make a basting sauce. After 30 minutes, lightly brush the top of the tofu slices with half of the sauce, and bake for another 15 minutes. Flip the slices and cook for another 30 minutes, then lightly brush the second side with more sauce and bake for another 15 minutes. The tofu should be chewy (not crunchy) and still very pliable.

3   Let the jerky cool completely (the slices will get a bit more crisp as they cool). Eat right away (or refrigerate in a sealed container for up to 1 week).

VARIATIONS

MISO JERKY   Swap miso paste for tomato paste, and skip the cumin and smoked paprika. Add ¼ teaspoon garlic powder if you'd like.

TERIYAKI JERKY   Use mirin instead of the tomato paste, ground ginger for the cumin, and onion powder for the smoked paprika.

GARLICKY TOFU JERKY   Add 1 teaspoon garlic powder along with the smoked paprika.

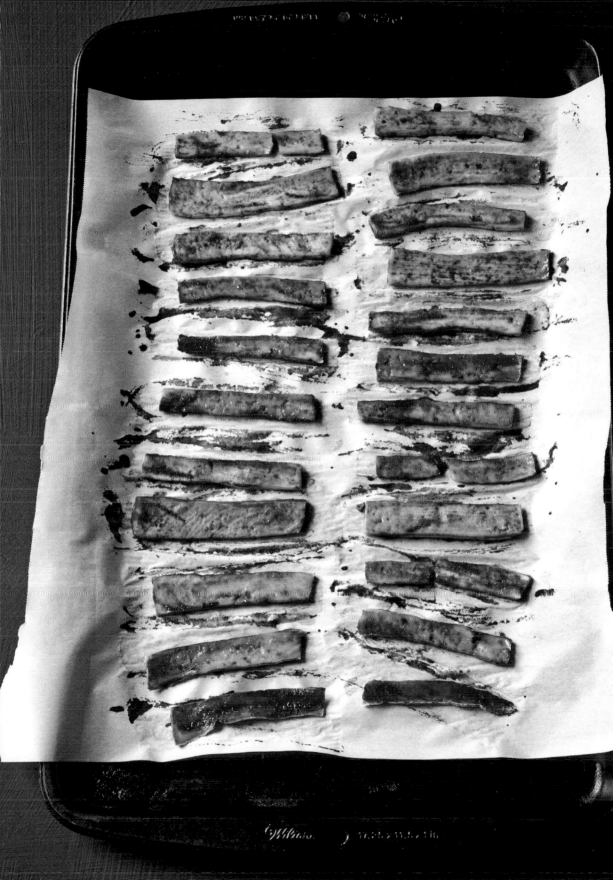

FRUIT CANDY

MAKES 4 servings   TIME 2 to 3½ hours, almost entirely unattended

Many packaged dried fruits are tossed in extra sugar and treated with preservatives, but you can avoid all that by oven-drying the fruit yourself. Though these "candies" are more calorie-dense than an equivalent weight of their raw counterparts—you are, after all, removing most of the water—they've still got all the fiber. And their intensity will satisfy even the most insistent sweet tooth.

About 1½ pounds fruit, like apple, pineapple, mango, banana, grapes, or strawberries

1 tablespoon olive oil

1   Heat the oven to 225°F. Peel the fruit, if necessary, and if they are already small (like berries or grapes), cut them in half; otherwise, cut them into wedges, sticks, or cubes about ¼ inch thick by 2 inches wide. Grease two baking sheets with the olive oil, then spread the fruit on the prepared pans in a single layer.

2   Cook the fruit until slightly shriveled, dehydrated, and sweet but still soft and chewy. You might have to move them or the pan around to ensure they don't burn or get too crisp. Start testing the fruit after about 2 hours, and remove it from the oven when it's as chewy or crisp as you like, anywhere from another 1 to 1½ hours depending on the fruit and how it was cut. Cool thoroughly before storing in an airtight container (they'll keep in the fridge for a week).

VARIATION

VEGETABLE CANDY The same technique works wonders on nearly any kind of vegetable. My favorites are green beans, asparagus, daikon, kohlrabi, sweet potatoes, and whole kale or chard leaves. Toss with ½ teaspoon salt and a bit of oil before slow-roasting. Vegetables will take somewhere between 2½ and 3 hours to dehydrate, depending on the cut and how dry they were to begin with.

MORE IDEAS

Almost any fruit will work with this recipe, including all berries, stone fruits, tropical fruits, even melons. Since there are no preservatives or conditioners involved the results for most will be darker than their commercial counterparts—more like roasted fruit.

FROZEN TROPICAL TRUFFLES

MAKES **4 servings**   TIME **20 minutes, plus time before and after for freezing**

Everyone needs a little sweet decadence now and then. These truffles take some advance planning, but they come together quickly and will keep beautifully in the freezer, ready when you are.

4 bananas, peeled

¼ cup unsweetened shredded coconut

¼ cup chopped pistachios

1 tablespoon maple syrup or other sweetener

1 tablespoon fresh lime juice

⅛ teaspoon salt

¼ cup cocoa powder

1 Mash the bananas in a medium bowl. Fold in the coconut, pistachios, syrup, lime juice, and salt with a rubber spatula until the ingredients are evenly distributed and the lumps are mostly smoothed out. Cover the bowl with plastic, pressing down on the banana mixture so there's no air between it and the plastic. Transfer the bowl to the freezer until the mixture is firm but not quite solid, 3 to 4 hours.

2 Put the cocoa on a small plate. Line a rimmed baking sheet with wax paper or parchment. With two spoons or your hands, shape the banana-coconut mixture into 16 balls (about 1½ inches in diameter; it's okay if they're not perfectly round); roll each in the cocoa powder and transfer to the prepared pan.

3 Put the pan in the freezer and freeze until the truffles are completely firm, 1 to 2 hours. Transfer them to an airtight container and serve frozen. (They'll keep for a month, but won't last that long!)

VARIATION

BANANA-PEANUT TRUFFLES A classic combination. Replace 1 banana with ¼ cup peanut butter and use ½ cup chopped roasted peanuts instead of the coconut and pistachios. Omit the lime juice. For a sweet and savory flavor, omit the maple syrup and increase the salt to ½ teaspoon.

MORE IDEAS

Toast the coconut first, for a more vibrant coconut flavor. • Use any nut instead of the pistachios. Cashews, hazelnuts, macadamias, or almonds would also be great here. • Instead of rolling in cocoa, dip the truffles in tempered dark chocolate (see the bonbons on page 210) and freeze the same way.

RASPBERRY SORBET ON A STICK

MAKES 4 servings   **TIME** 10 minutes, plus 2 hours to freeze

You have a choice here: You can use packaged (unsweetened) frozen fruit—a boon in the dead of winter—or you can cut and freeze fresh fruit before getting started. Either molds or paper cups and wooden sticks will work—anything in that 4- to 6-ounce range.

2 cups fresh or frozen raspberries

2 teaspoons fresh lemon juice

2 tablespoons maple syrup or other sweetener (optional)

1   Put the fruit, lemon juice, and maple syrup, if you're using it, in a food processor. Add 1 tablespoon of water and puree until smooth, stopping the machine to scrape down the sides once or twice. Add more water, 1 tablespoon at a time, to keep the machine working, being careful not to overprocess and turn the fruit to juice.

2   Spoon the sorbet into plastic molds or small paper cups arranged on a tray, and transfer them to the freezer. If they don't already have sticks, after an hour or so, insert one into each cup, and freeze until solid.

3   To remove the pops, run them upside down under cool water for a few seconds and loosen them from the mold.

VARIATIONS

PIÑA COLADA ON A STICK Use pineapple for the fruit and add ¼ cup unsweetened shredded coconut, 2 tablespoons coconut milk (reduced-fat is fine), and some fresh mint before pureeing.

THAI ICED TEA ON A STICK Combine 2 cups black tea, ½ cup coconut milk (reduced-fat is fine), and 1 teaspoon five-spice powder or cinnamon to the mix.

MELON-CUCUMBER ON A STICK Instead of raspberries try 1 cup chopped melon (any kind) and 1 cup chopped cucumber. Add ¼ cup fresh lime juice and ¼ cup fresh cilantro before pureeing.

SPICY MANGO ON A STICK Skip the sweetener. Use 2 cups chopped mango instead of the raspberries and lime juice instead of the lemon juice. Add some or all of a fresh hot red chile (like Thai or serrano), or ¼ teaspoon cayenne, before processing.

MORE IDEAS

I hope it's obvious you can use any fruit you like here. Chop it up as needed. • Go savory: Skip the sweetener and add a pinch of sea salt and a few grinds of pepper, and use more lemon juice instead of the water. • Add chocolate. Make sure it's good-quality dark chocolate; 1 or 2 ounces per batch is plenty. Chop it fine and add it after pureeing the fruit in Step 1. • Add fresh herbs to the pops: Figure about 2 tablespoons for each batch. • Replace the water with other liquids, like coffee, tea, or non-dairy milk.

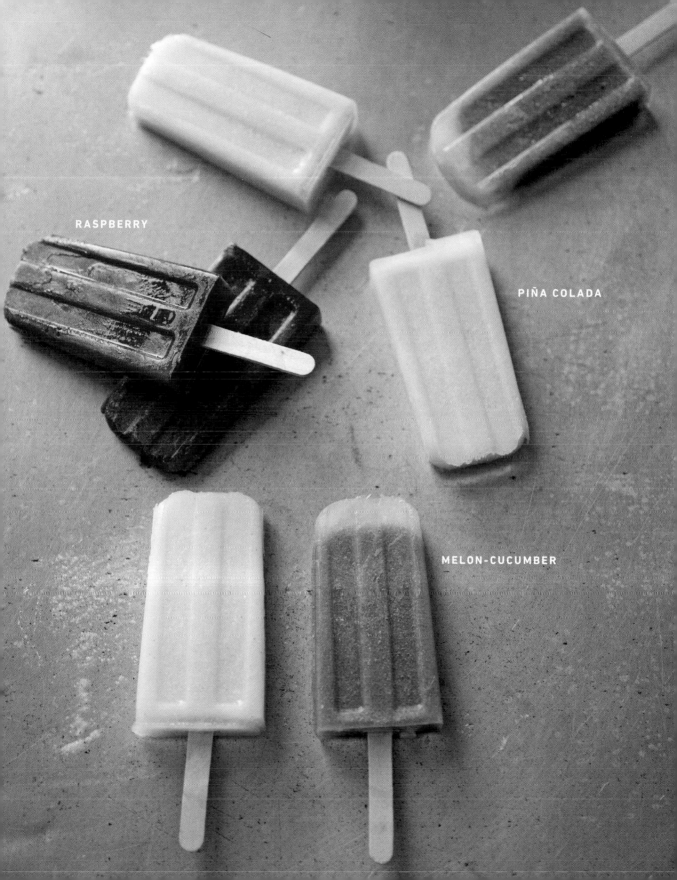

RASPBERRY

PIÑA COLADA

MELON-CUCUMBER

DINNER

SUCCOTASH PASTA

RISOTTO WITH BRUSSELS
SPROUTS

PANE COTTO

JÍCAMA SALAD WITH
SALMON STEAKS

FISH WITH VEGETABLE GRATIN

RED PAELLA WITH SCALLOPS

BEANS, SHRIMP, AND FENNEL

MUSSELS IN COCONUT BROTH

CHICKEN STIR-FRY IN
LETTUCE CUPS

CHICKEN WITH FENNEL SALAD

GINGERED RICE WITH CHICKEN

JERK CHICKEN BURGERS

CHICKEN VEGETABLE TAGINE

AFRICAN-STYLE CHICKEN STEW

PROVENÇAL CHICKEN STEW

GINGERY WINTER STEW

PORK, ASPARAGUS, AND SOBA

CRISP PORK ON GREEN PAPAYA
SALAD

PORK CHOP PAN ROAST

HAM HASH WITH GREENS

SWEET POTATO SHEPHERD'S PIE

BÁNH MÌ MEATBALL SALAD

SCHEZUAN BEEF AND CELERY

STEAK AU POIVRE WITH
MUSHROOMS

GRITS AND GRILLADES

VEGETABLE CURRY WITH LAMB

When six o'clock rolls around it's time for the evening meal. Whether you dine in a fine restaurant, gather around the table with family, or sit alone in front of the television with a bowl of pasta, you should always focus on relaxing and enjoying—both the anticipation and the eating—rather than fretting about your diet.

That's what makes VB6 sustainable and successful: The lessons learned throughout the day will almost certainly carry over to your after-six choices.

The dinners here are not blowout meals loaded with treats. Instead these are examples of "flexitarian" eating: main dishes that include moderate amounts of meat, poultry, fish, or dairy, and that use those ingredients in a supporting role to accompany vegetables, grains, and legumes.

When you eat the Standard American Diet, it's too easy to forget that meat is a luxury and that plants are not only the basis of a good human diet, but a pleasure. The recipes in this chapter are for familiar, easy-to-prepare dishes that will help you re-balance the way you approach dinner. They're loaded with variations and ideas to help inspire a lifetime of good eating.

VB6 dinners aren't about self-deprivation or even drastic change, but rather the benefits that come from some simple readjustments. Soon you won't need an 8-ounce steak to satisfy you; 2 to 3 ounces will do the trick. And you'll find that only rarely will animal foods be at the center of the meal anymore, even when cooking for guests. After a day of plant-based eating, you'll notice—and deeply appreciate—the flavor and texture of even a small pat of butter or a crumble of bacon or sausage. And it'll make you glad.

SUCCOTASH PASTA

MAKES 4 servings   **TIME** 30 minutes

Some people shy away from eating starch with pasta, but there are loads of classic dishes that combine noodles with potatoes or beans. And there's so much else going on here—texture, color, flavor—why worry? For this dish to work best, try to chop all the vegetables the size of the corn or no larger than the beans so things cook evenly. And be sure to see the variations; once you start playing around with this style of dish, you'll find that the possibilities are endless.

1½ teaspoons salt

8 ounces any cut pasta, preferably whole wheat

2 ears fresh corn

3 tablespoons olive oil

1 summer squash or zucchini, chopped

¼ teaspoon pepper

1 bunch scallions, white and green parts separated and chopped

1 tablespoon minced garlic

2 large tomatoes, chopped

2 cups fresh or frozen lima beans

1 cup grated Parmesan cheese

1 cup chopped fresh basil

1   Bring a large pot of water to a boil and add 1 teaspoon salt. Cook the pasta, stirring occasionally, until it's tender but not mushy; start tasting for doneness after 5 minutes.

2   Meanwhile, husk the corn. Carefully cut the kernels from the cobs with a sharp knife, slicing away from you; save as much of their juice as you can. Put 1 tablespoon of the oil in a large skillet over medium-high heat. Add the corn and cook, stirring occasionally, until the kernels are browned in places, 2 to 3 minutes. Transfer to a plate.

3   Return the pan to the heat and add another tablespoon of the oil and the summer squash; sprinkle with the remaining ½ teaspoon salt and the pepper. Cook, stirring occasionally and adjusting the heat as necessary, until the squash softens and the pan is almost dry again, 3 to 5 minutes. Transfer to the plate with the corn and return the pan to medium heat.

4   Add the remaining 1 tablespoon oil to the skillet with the white parts of the scallion and the garlic. Cook, stirring occasionally, until the vegetables soften and are translucent, 1 or 2 minutes. Add the tomatoes and lima beans and cook, stirring, until the tomatoes are just hot and beginning to ooze some juice; turn off the heat.

5   When the pasta is ready, drain it, reserving some of the cooking water. Add the pasta to the skillet along with the corn and squash and turn the heat to high. Cook no more than 1 minute, stirring constantly and adding just enough of the reserved cooking water to heat the pasta and make a sauce. Remove from the heat, add the scallion greens, the Parmesan, and basil, and serve.

SUCCOTASH WITH SHRIMP Really no more than a shrimp stir-fry. Skip the pasta, so don't bother to put a pot of water on to boil in Step 1. Have 1 pound peeled shrimp handy. After you cook the corn in the oil in Step 2, add the shrimp and keep stirring until it's pink and slightly firm, just 1 or 2 minutes more. Then follow the recipe and serve over brown rice or a bed of greens.

PUMPKIN PASTA For the fall or winter when succotash ingredients aren't in their prime, use 1 bunch chopped Swiss chard instead of the corn. Substitute pumpkin for the summer squash: peel and seed it, and cut it into 1-inch cubes. Use a 14-ounce can of diced tomatoes and their juice instead of the fresh tomatoes, and garnish with fresh parsley (or nothing) instead of the basil.

MORE IDEAS

Instead of lima beans, try other frozen beans, like fava beans, black-eyed peas, edamame, or even peas. • Eggplant is an easy alternative to summer squash. Chop and cook it the same way. • Instead of garnishing with scallions, try fresh cilantro and a squeeze of lime or lemon. Then serve the dish at room temperature or lightly chilled, like a pasta salad.

MAKING DINNERS VEGAN

All of the recipes in this chapter are easy to adjust so that they contain no animal foods, so you can make whatever adjustments in your eating day you'd like. Here's how:

- Replace cheese with chopped nuts or seeds.

- A spoonful of silken tofu is a nice substitute for eggs; or you can just toss cooked or canned beans into the dish; heat just long enough to warm through.

- Instead of roasted, grilled, or broiled meat, fish, or poultry, try cooking firm tofu slices the same way; cut a block crosswise no more than 1 inch thick. It might take a little longer to brown; it's ready to turn when it releases easily from the pan.

- For stir-fries, replace the meat with crumbled tofu or tempeh. Or add frozen beans—like lima, fava, or edamame—to the vegetables toward the end of cooking.

- Burgers are a little trickier, but doable. Substitute beans for the weight of the meat, then pulse them in the food processor a few times just until a pinch sticks together. Mix in the other ingredients. Cook under the broiler—not on the grill.

RISOTTO WITH
BRUSSELS SPROUTS

MAKES 4 servings   TIME About 45 minutes

After eating vegetables all day, even a little bit of butter and cheese feels
rich and indulgent. I put mine to good use in a semi-classic risotto. It may
take you some time to come around to brown rice in this dish, but find a
good short-grain variety and you will start to crave it.

1½ teaspoons salt

1½ cups short- or
medium-grain brown rice

2 tablespoons olive oil

1 onion, chopped

1 tablespoon minced garlic

½ teaspoon pepper

Zest of 1 lemon

½ cup dry white wine
(optional)

2 cups chicken or vegetable
stock (see page 246), or
water, plus more as needed

1 pound Brussels sprouts,
chopped

½ cup grated Parmesan
cheese

½ cup crumbled Gorgonzola
cheese

1 tablespoon butter

2 teaspoons fresh lemon
juice

1 Bring about 6 cups water and 1 teaspoon salt to a boil in a large pot.
Stir in the rice, adjust the heat so that the water bubbles steadily, and
cook, undisturbed, until the rice is plump and partially tender, 10 to
15 minutes. Drain well, reserving the cooking water.

2 Put the oil in a large skillet over medium heat. Add the onion and
garlic, and cook, stirring occasionally, until the vegetables soften, 3 to
5 minutes. Add the rice and cook, stirring occasionally, until it is glossy
and coated with oil, 2 to 3 minutes. Add the remaining ½ teaspoon salt
and the pepper and zest, then the wine if you're using it (or ½ cup of the
stock or reserved cooking water). Stir and let the liquid bubble away.

3 Begin adding the stock or the reserved rice-cooking water ½ cup or
so at a time, stirring after each addition. When the liquid is just about
absorbed, add more. (If you're using stock, add it all before starting
with the cooking water; if you run out of cooking water, switch to warm
tap water.) The mixture should be neither soupy nor dry. Keep the heat
at medium to medium-high and stir frequently. Begin tasting the rice
10 minutes after you add it; you want it to be barely tender, still with a
bit of crunch; it could take as long as 20 minutes to reach this stage.
When it does, add the Brussels sprouts.

4 Cook, stirring and adding just enough liquid to prevent the rice from
sticking, until the Brussels sprouts soften and turn bright green, 3 to
5 minutes. Add the cheeses, butter, and lemon juice and keep stirring
until they melt. Taste and adjust the seasoning and serve right away.

RISOTTO WITH CHARRED BRUSSELS SPROUTS For a more assertive smoky flavor, heat the broiler. Toss the chopped Brussels sprouts with an additional tablespoon of olive oil and spread them on a large rimmed baking sheet. Broil, turning several times and watching them like a hawk, until they're bright green and dark in places. Stir them into the rice with the cheeses in Step 4.

RISOTTO WITH BRUSSELS SPROUTS AND FIGS A little sweetness works surprisingly well here. Slice 1 pint black or green fresh figs, or soak ½ cup chopped dried figs in 1 cup boiling water for 5 minutes; if using dried, drain them, reserving the steeping liquid to incorporate into the risotto instead of some of the stock. Add the reconstituted figs with the Brussels sprouts in Step 3; if using fresh, add them with the cheeses in Step 4.

MORE IDEAS

Instead of brown rice, you can make a more traditional risotto by using Arborio, Carnaroli, Vialone, or Nano rice. Don't parboil it; proceed directly to Step 2. The total cooking time in Step 3 could be as long at 30 minutes.
• Instead of Brussels sprouts, you can use fresh or frozen corn kernels, chopped broccoli or cauliflower, or any kind of cabbage or kale.

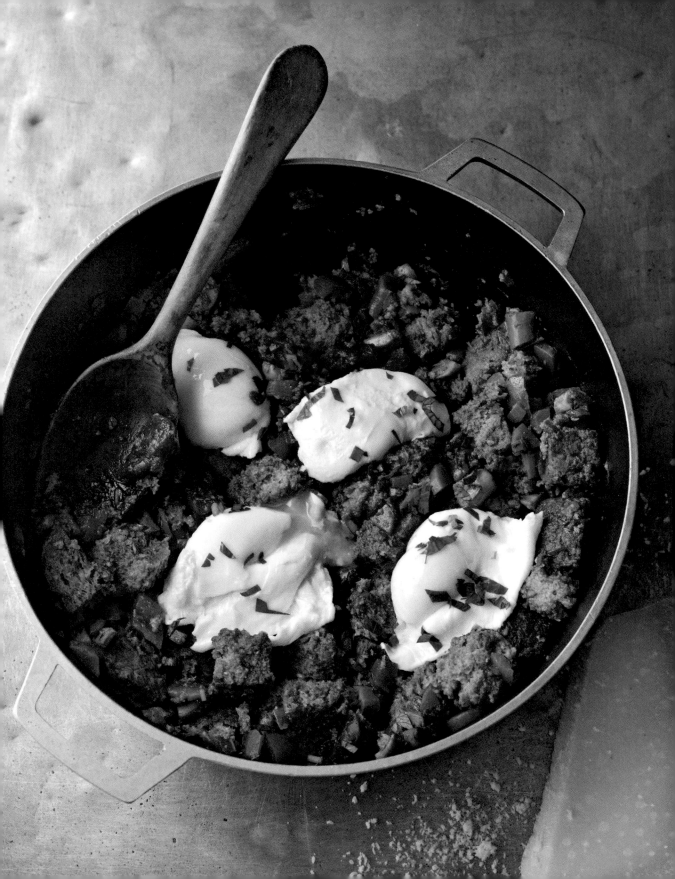

PANE COTTO

MAKES 4 servings   **TIME** About 90 minutes

I love the strangely pleasant texture of bread after it sits in flavorful liquid. "Cooked bread" (literally) and its cousins *panzanella* and *papa pomodoro* are part of a family of classic Italian recipes that work this simple magic. Use pane cotto as a base for poaching eggs, and it quickly becomes a one-dish meal. Add a salad, and you're all set. To make this in the oven, or for a larger group, see the variations that follow.

4 thick slices whole-grain bread (stale is fine), cubed

3 tablespoons olive oil

1 pound button mushrooms, chopped

1 onion, chopped

1 tablespoon minced garlic

2 carrots, chopped

1 red or green bell pepper, chopped

1 teaspoon salt

½ teaspoon pepper

One 28-ounce can diced tomatoes with their juice

4 eggs

½ cup grated Parmesan cheese

½ cup chopped fresh basil, or ¼ cup chopped fresh parsley (optional)

1 Heat the oven to 400°F. Put the bread on a baking sheet and toast, turning once or twice, until golden and dry, 10 to 15 minutes. Remove the bread from the oven as soon as it's ready.

2 Meanwhile, put the oil in a large pot over medium heat. When it's hot, add the mushrooms and cook, stirring occasionally, until they release their liquid and the pan is becoming dry again, 3 to 5 minutes. Add the onion and garlic and cook, stirring until they become fragrant, just 1 or 2 minutes. Then add the carrots and bell pepper, and sprinkle with the salt and pepper. Cook, stirring occasionally, until the carrots and bell pepper start to get soft, 3 to 5 minutes.

3 Add the tomatoes, bring the sauce to a boil, then adjust the heat so it bubbles steadily. Cook, stirring occasionally, until the tomatoes break down, the vegetables become very soft, and the mixture thickens, 10 to 15 minutes.

4 Add the bread and stir to coat it with the sauce. If the mixture looks too thick or is sticking to the pan, stir in a splash of water—you want it to be about the consistency of thick soup. Taste and adjust the seasoning. Bring to a gentle bubble, make indentations with the back of a spoon for the eggs, then crack them into the pan. Cover and simmer until eggs are as soft or as firm as you like them, 2 to 5 minutes.

5 Scatter the cheese on top, followed by the basil or parsley, if using it, and serve.

(recipe continues)

BAKED PANE COTTO Another way to set the eggs is by baking them. After the toast comes out of the oven, lower the heat to 350°F. In Step 4, once the eggs are added to the skillet, sprinkle the cheese over all and pop the pan in the oven to cook until the eggs are set how you like them, 10 to 20 minutes. Then garnish with the herb and serve.

BAKED PANE COTTO FOR A CROWD The easiest ever. Double the bread and sauce ingredients and make both the bread and sauce components up to a day ahead if you like. Heat the oven to 350°F. Spread the mixture into a 9 by 13-inch baking dish, make the indentations, add the eggs, top with the cheese, and bake as above. (It will take 5 to 10 minutes longer if the dish goes into the oven cold.)

MORE IDEAS

If you don't have fresh herbs, season the sauce with up to 2 teaspoons dried oregano or thyme. • Crank up the heat by adding a small fresh hot chile or a pinch of red chile flakes along with the bell pepper. • Explore different vegetables, like fennel. • Use red or white wine instead of water to thin the sauce before adding the eggs. • Try crumbled ricotta salata or Gorgonzola cheese instead of the Parmesan.

JÍCAMA SALAD WITH SALMON STEAKS

MAKES 4 servings   **TIME** 40 minutes

With its assertive flavor and rich texture, salmon benefits from bright and refreshing companions. Enter this light, crisp salad. I like salmon steaks here since they're sturdy enough for grilling or broiling, but skin-on fillets are fine too.

1 jícama, chopped (about 2 cups)

½ large pineapple, chopped (about 2 cups)

1 red bell pepper, chopped

4 scallions, sliced

¼ cup chopped fresh mint

3 tablespoons fresh lime juice

3 tablespoons olive oil

1 teaspoon salt

Pinch cayenne (optional)

4 salmon steaks, preferably wild (about 1½ pounds)

½ teaspoon pepper

1   Prepare a grill or turn on the broiler; put the rack 4 inches from the heat source. Combine the jícama, pineapple, bell pepper, scallions, mint, lime juice, and 2 tablespoons olive oil in a large bowl. Sprinkle with half the salt and the cayenne, if you're using it; toss, taste and adjust the seasoning, toss again, and let sit in the fridge for at least 10 minutes or up to a few hours.

2   Drizzle the fish with the remaining 1 tablespoon olive oil and sprinkle it with the remaining ½ teaspoon salt and the pepper. When the grill or broiler is hot, put the salmon on the hot grill or on a rimmed baking sheet under the broiler and cook, turning once, until browned and just cooked through, 3 to 4 minutes per side. (When they're ready, a thin-bladed knife will pass through the flesh fairly easily.)

3   To serve, toss the vegetables one last time and divide among shallow bowls. Serve the fish on top of the salad.

VARIATION

FISH TACOS WITH JÍCAMA SLAW Instead of serving this dish as an elegant steak-and-salad combo, you can easily turn it into a more casual fish taco. Warm 8 to 12 corn tortillas. Instead of chopping the pineapple and vegetables in Step 1, slice them into thin shreds (or grate them). After cooking the fish, break it into pieces, discarding the skin and bones, and tuck it into the tortillas. Top with some of the salad and serve, passing the rest at the table.

MORE IDEAS

If you can't find good wild salmon, use 4 boneless trout fillets or look for Arctic char; farm-raised salmon is fine too. If you don't like salmon, grill any sturdy fish, or opt for shrimp or scallops. • Radishes are a good substitute for jícama. Figure 2 bunches small radishes or 1 daikon. • Try red onion or shallots instead of scallions. • Try cilantro, dill, or Thai basil instead of the mint in the salad.

FISH WITH VEGETABLE GRATIN

MAKES 4 servings   **TIME** 40 minutes, largely unattended

Here's a way to cook an entire meal at once, simply by taking advantage of a hot oven; it's a boon for easy entertaining or busy weeknights. You can use just about any fish fillets you like—halibut, catfish, salmon, bass, or char are all good choices; even shrimp or scallops work well baked in a package like this. And the recipe is really very easy to multiply and cook for a crowd.

4 tablespoons olive oil

2 zucchini, thinly sliced crosswise

1 pound asparagus (thick ends peeled if you like), sliced into 1-inch pieces

2 tomatoes, thinly sliced crosswise

1 onion, sliced crosswise and separated into rings

4 (or more) whole garlic cloves

1 teaspoon salt

½ teaspoon pepper

1 cup whole wheat breadcrumbs (see page 251)

About 1 pound thick white fish fillets (see headnote)

Juice of 1 lemon

¼ cup chopped fresh parsley, for garnish

Lemon wedges

1   Heat the oven to 400°F and arrange the racks so you have room for two pans. Grease a 2-quart baking dish or a 9 by 13-inch baking pan with 1 tablespoon oil. Layer the zucchini, asparagus, tomatoes, and onion in the prepared dish (in that order); tuck in the garlic here and there. Sprinkle with half the salt and pepper, cover with foil, and bake until the vegetables are tender and releasing their juices, 15 to 20 minutes.

2   Uncover the gratin, sprinkle with breadcrumbs, and drizzle with 2 tablespoons oil. Continue baking until the vegetables are nearly dry and the breadcrumbs have toasted, 25 to 30 minutes.

3   Meanwhile, put the fish on a big piece of foil in a rimmed baking sheet. Sprinkle with the remaining ½ teaspoon salt and ¼ teaspoon pepper and drizzle with the remaining 1 tablespoon oil, then drizzle the lemon juice over all. Cover with another piece of foil and crimp the edges to seal. About 10 minutes into the second baking time for the gratin, add the pan with the fish to the oven. Cook undisturbed until a knife tip inserted through the foil into the fish meets with no resistance, 10 to 15 minutes (or if you happen to notice, about 8 minutes from when the fish begins sizzling). If the vegetables are ready before the fish is, remove them from the oven.

4   Cut into the top of the foil fish packet, opening it carefully so that the steam escapes away from you. Serve the fish drizzled with its pan juices, alongside the vegetables and garnished with the parsley. Serve with lemon wedges.

BAKED CHICKEN WITH VEGETABLE GRATIN Essentially poached chicken. Use boneless breasts or thighs instead of the fish. The breasts will be done in about the same time; figure another 5 to 10 minutes for chicken thighs.

BAKED FISH WITH SWEET POTATO GRATIN Peel and slice 2 pounds sweet potatoes. Omit the breadcrumbs if you'd like. In Step 1, the potatoes will take longer than the mixed vegetables to become tender and won't release water, so leave them covered until you can easily slip a sharp knife into the center of the baking dish, 40 to 50 minutes. Then uncover, drizzle with the oil, and keep baking until the top is golden, another 15 to 20 minutes. For an excellent holiday side dish, skip the fish entirely.

MORE IDEAS

Of course, many foods that can be baked can also be grilled. If you've got a hankering, prepare a charcoal or gas grill for the fish—or whatever meat or poultry you choose. • Add a couple of fresh thyme sprigs or bay leaves to the foil package before sealing and baking it. • Other vegetables to try in the gratin are eggplant, fennel, bell peppers, and broccoli or cauliflower florets. • This gratin is great on its own—for lunch or as a side for simply cooked roasts, beans, or grains.

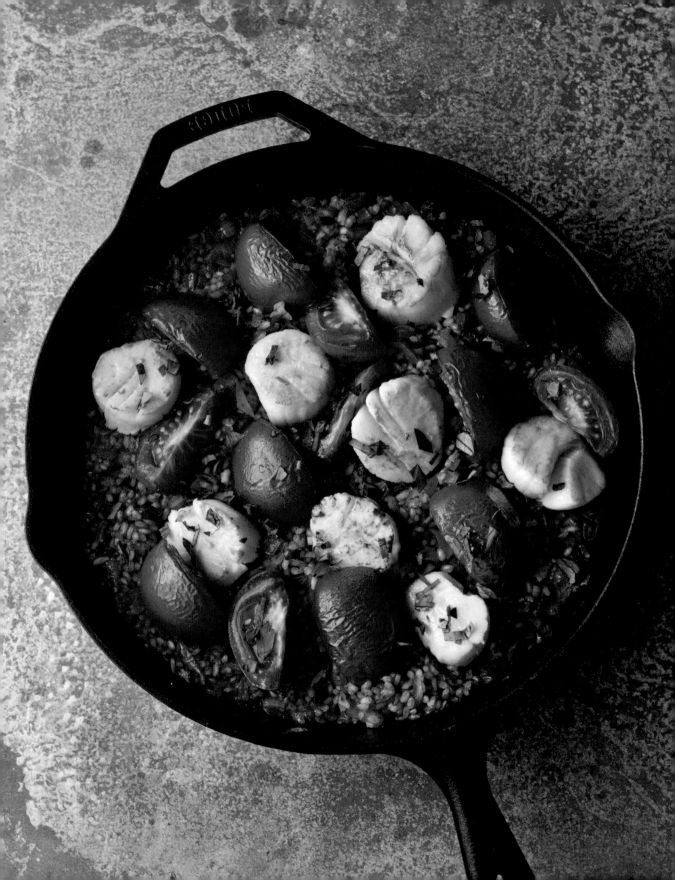

RED PAELLA WITH SCALLOPS

MAKES 4 servings   **TIME** 50 minutes

A streamlined paella, loaded with vegetables and flavored like the sea.
Parboiling gives brown rice a head start and helps the kernels absorb
liquid quickly in the oven. Tomatoes balance the sweetness of the scallops
and the smokiness of the spice here perfectly. You can use any kind of
tomato—even whole cherry tomatoes if that's what you like—so choose
whatever's ripest.

2 teaspoons salt

1½ cups short-grain brown
rice

1 pound tomatoes, cut into
thick wedges

4 tablespoons olive oil

1 pound sea scallops

½ teaspoon pepper

1 onion, chopped

1 tablespoon minced garlic

1 tablespoon tomato paste

1 tablespoon smoked
paprika

2 cups fish or vegetable
stock (see page 246), or
water, plus more as needed

¼ cup chopped fresh
parsley, for garnish

Lemon wedges

1 Heat the oven to 450°F. Bring a medium pot of water and 1 teaspoon
salt to a boil. Stir in the rice, adjust the heat so that the water bubbles
steadily, and cook undisturbed until the rice is plump and partially
tender, 10 to 15 minutes. Drain well. Put the tomatoes in a medium
bowl, sprinkle with ½ teaspoon of salt, and drizzle with 1 tablespoon of
the olive oil. Toss gently.

2 Put 2 tablespoons of the oil in a 10- or 12-inch ovenproof skillet
over medium-high heat. Pat the scallops dry with paper towels, add
them to the pan, and sprinkle with the remaining ½ teaspoon salt and
the pepper; work in batches if necessary to avoid crowding the skillet.
Cook, turning once, until the scallops are browned on both sides and
just cooked through, 1 to 3 minutes per side depending on how thick
they are. Transfer them to a plate.

3 Put the remaining 1 tablespoon oil in the same skillet over medium-
high heat. Add the onion and garlic and cook, stirring occasionally,
until the vegetables soften, 3 to 5 minutes. Stir in the tomato paste and
paprika and cook until fragrant, no more than 1 minute. Add the rice
and cook, stirring occasionally, until it's shiny, another 1 or 2 minutes.
Carefully add the stock and stir until just combined.

4 Put the tomatoes on top of the rice and drizzle with the juices that
accumulated in the bottom of the bowl. Transfer the pan to the oven
and cook undisturbed for 15 minutes. Test a kernel of rice. If it's not
quite tender and the pan looks too dry, add a small amount of stock
and return it to the oven; if it's not tender and the pan looks soupy, just
return it to the oven. Check again in another 5 minutes.

5 When the rice is ready, nestle the scallops in among the tomatoes,
return the pan to the oven, and turn off the heat. Let the paella sit
until the scallops are heated through, 2 or 3 minutes. Garnish with the
parsley and serve with lemon wedges.

(recipe continues)

RED PAELLA WITH SCALLOPS CON SOCCARRAT You know those crisp bits of rice around the edge and bottom of the pan? This is how you get them: After the paella rests in Step 4, put the pan over high heat for a few minutes to develop a bit of a crust; adjust the heat so it sizzles but doesn't burn, and stop the minute the paella starts to smell like toast.

RED PAELLA WITH SCALLOPS AND CHORIZO Reduce the scallops to 12 ounces. Add 4 ounces chopped chorizo in Step 3 along with the onion and garlic. Cook, stirring occasionally, until the fat releases and the chorizo browns a bit, then stir in the tomato paste and proceed with the recipe.

CURRIED PAELLA WITH SCALLOPS It's remarkable how one small switch can make such a difference. Substitute curry powder for the smoked paprika.

MORE IDEAS

Instead of the tomatoes, you've got a couple of options. Zucchini and eggplant can both be treated the same way, for example. • For the scallops, try substituting shrimp or squid, or strips of chicken thighs, beef sirloin, or pork loin.
• Instead of the smoked paprika, use a pinch of saffron threads.

BEANS, SHRIMP, AND FENNEL

MAKES 4 servings   TIME 25 minutes

If you've never tried this combination, do. Like now. Beans with seafood is not only just as classic but also just as tasty as beans with pork.
(And it's faster.) You control the texture here: The main recipe results in
creamy beans in a thick broth; but see the variations for a drier stir-fry
and a tomato, shrimp, and bean stew.

4 cups cooked or canned
white beans (see page 232)

3 tablespoons olive oil

1 onion, halved and sliced

1 teaspoon salt

½ teaspoon pepper

1 pound fennel, bulb
trimmed and thinly sliced

1 tablespoon minced garlic

2 bay leaves

2 cups vegetable or chicken
stock (see page 246), or
water, plus more as needed

1 pound peeled shrimp

2 tablespoons fresh lemon
juice

1 tablespoon chopped fresh
oregano or marjoram

1   Drain the beans. If you made them yourself, reserve the cooking
liquid; if they're canned, discard it and rinse the beans. Put the oil in a
large skillet over medium heat. When it's hot, add the onion, sprinkle
with the salt and pepper, and cook, stirring occasionally, until it softens
and turns golden, 3 to 5 minutes. Add the fennel, garlic, and bay leaves;
continue cooking and stirring until fragrant, 1 or 2 minutes more.

2   Add the beans to the pot along with a total of 2 cups liquid, either the
bean-cooking liquid, stock, water, or a combination. Bring the mixture
to a boil, then lower the heat so it bubbles steadily and cook, stirring
occasionally until the beans and vegetables become quite tender, 10 to
15 minutes. If you'd like, mash some of the beans with the spoon to help
thicken the sauce; add more liquid if the mixture ever looks too dry.

3   When the beans are the texture you like, add the shrimp and cover
the pot. Cook, stirring once or twice, just until the shrimp turn opaque,
3 to 5 minutes. Add the lemon juice and herb, taste and adjust the
seasoning, and serve.

VARIATIONS

STIR-FRIED WHITE BEANS WITH SHRIMP AND FENNEL   Nice party
food spooned over thin slices of toasted baguette, crostini style. In
Step 1, cook the fennel and onion until they're golden and almost silky,
another 5 minutes or so. When you add the beans in Step 2, add the
shrimp too; when the shrimp are done, the beans will be hot. Season
and serve as described at the end of Step 3.

WHITE BEANS AND SHRIMP, BOUILLABAISSE STYLE   Instead of
the onion, use two well-rinsed sliced leeks and increase the liquid to
4 cups. In Step 2, add one 28-ounce can diced tomatoes and a big pinch
of saffron. Bring the stew to a boil, then adjust the heat so it bubbles
steadily and cook, stirring occasionally, until the beans thicken the
broth and the tomatoes break down, 10 to 15 minutes. Add the shrimp,
then cook and season as directed in Step 3. Remove the bay leaves, put
2 slices of baguette in each bowl, and ladle the stew on top.

MUSSELS IN COCONUT BROTH

MAKES 4 servings   **TIME** 30 minutes

A bountiful bowl—filled with vegetables, seafood, and noodles—that's
so big you might think you'll have trouble finishing it, but trust me: You
won't leave a drop behind.

2 tablespoons vegetable oil

1 tablespoon minced ginger

1 tablespoon minced garlic

1 (or more) fresh or dried
green or red chiles

2 lemongrass stalks, cut
into 3-inch pieces

4 tablespoons fresh lime
juice

1 teaspoon salt

½ teaspoon pepper

12 ounces thin brown rice
noodles or whole wheat
angel hair

½ cup coconut milk
(reduced-fat is fine)

4 ounces daikon, peeled and
chopped

1 red bell pepper, sliced

1 carrot, cut into coins

3 pounds mussels,
preferably wild, well
scrubbed

2 scallions, sliced

½ cup chopped fresh
cilantro, for garnish

1   Bring a kettle of water to a boil. Put 1 tablespoon oil in a large pot over medium heat. Add the ginger and garlic and cook, stirring occasionally, until they puff and begin to soften, about 1 minute. Add the chiles, lemongrass, lime juice, salt, and pepper to the pot along with 2 cups water. Cook, stirring occasionally and adjusting the heat as necessary so the mixture bubbles steadily, 3 to 5 minutes.

2   When the kettle comes to a boil, put the noodles in a large heatproof bowl and cover with boiling water. Let sit, stirring once or twice with a fork, until the noodles are tender but not mushy, 3 to 5 minutes. Drain well and toss with the remaining 1 tablespoon oil.

3   Add the coconut milk to the pot along with the daikon, bell pepper, and carrot; stir and return the liquid to a bubble. Carefully put the mussels on top of the vegetables, sprinkle with the scallions, turn the heat up to high, and cover the pot. Cook, shaking the pot occasionally, until all (or nearly all) of the shells open, 5 to 10 minutes. (Discard any that do not open.)

4   Divide the noodles among shallow bowls. Ladle the mussels, vegetables, and broth over the rice noodles, fishing out the lemongrass stalks as you see them. Garnish with the cilantro and serve.

VARIATIONS

MUSSELS, CORN, AND NOODLES IN COCONUT BROTH Unreal with fresh corn on the cob, but when it isn't in season, 2 cups frozen kernels is a fine substitute. Skip the daikon. Husk 2 ears of corn and cut the cobs crosswise into coins about 1 inch wide. Toss them into the pot with the coconut milk and other vegetables in Step 3.

MUSSELS, VEGETABLES, AND PASTA IN TOMATO BROTH You can take this in a completely different direction by swapping a few key ingredients. Substitute olive oil for the vegetable oil, another tablespoon of minced garlic for the ginger, 4 bay leaves for the lemongrass, 2 cups chopped tomatoes instead of the water, and chopped fresh basil instead of the cilantro. For the vegetables, try 1 bunch chopped escarole and use angel hair (whole wheat is nice) instead of the rice noodles.

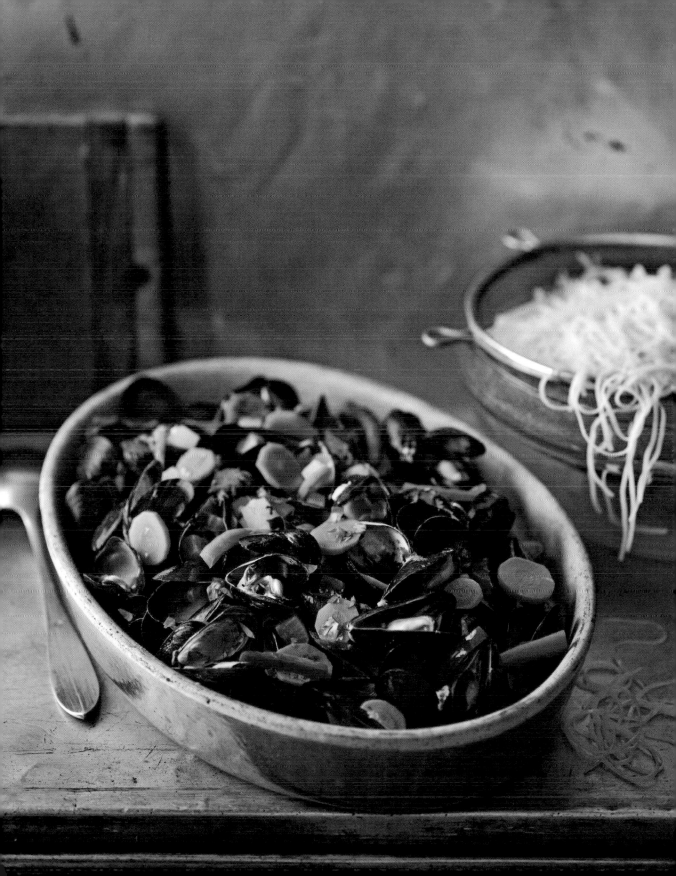

CHICKEN STIR-FRY IN LETTUCE CUPS

MAKES 4 servings   **TIME** 40 minutes

Wrappers are a great way to turn a stir-fry into something fun and inter-active for entertaining, or for an ultra-casual supper. Here are some tips: Iceberg and Bibb (or Boston) lettuce leaves are naturally cupped to hold fillings; broad-leafed and sturdy green and red leaf lettuces are better if you want to enfold the filling like burritos. I prefer to let everyone assemble his or her own, but you can certainly do it for your guests—just not too far in advance or the leaves will get soggy. For the easiest eating, make sure to chop the chicken and vegetables about the same size; ½ inch or so is ideal.

1 head iceberg, Bibb, or other lettuce

2 tablespoons vegetable oil

12 ounces boneless, skinless chicken thighs, chopped

½ teaspoon salt

½ teaspoon pepper

2 tablespoons minced garlic

1 tablespoon minced ginger

1 bunch scallions, green and white parts separated, chopped

1 carrot, chopped

½ pound asparagus (thick ends peeled if you like) or snow peas, chopped

½ pound shiitake mushrooms, chopped

2 celery stalks, chopped

¼ cup chicken or vegetable stock (see page 246), or water

2 tablespoons soy sauce

1 Core the lettuce and, working from the outside in, carefully remove as many intact leaves as you can. Rinse and wrap them in towels and refrigerate for up to several hours in advance.

2 Put a large skillet over high heat. Add 1 tablespoon oil, swirl it around, and immediately add the chicken, sprinkling it with the salt and pepper. Cook undisturbed until the pieces brown and release from the pan easily. Then add the garlic and ginger, and stir frequently until the chicken is no longer pink and the vegetables soften, 3 to 5 minutes total. Remove the meat mixture from the pan.

3 Add the remaining 1 tablespoon oil along with the white parts of the scallions, and cook, stirring occasionally and adjusting the heat to avoid burning, until they turn golden, 2 or 3 minutes. Add remaining vegetables (except the scallion greens) one at a time and stirring between each addition; cook until they're crisp-tender, no more than 5 minutes total.

4 Return the chicken mixture to the pan along with the stock, soy sauce, and scallion greens. Cook and stir, scraping up any browned bits from the bottom of the skillet and adding just enough more stock to help the mixture make a little sauce, just 1 minute more. Turn off the heat.

5 Whisk the mayonnaise, lime juice, and sriracha with ¼ cup water. Taste and adjust the seasoning, adding more lime or hot sauce as you like. Serve the chicken and vegetables with the lettuce leaves for wrapping (or filling), with the sauce alongside for dipping.

EDAMAME AND VEGETABLES IN LETTUCE CUPS Use 3 cups frozen edamame instead of the chicken. No need to thaw the beans first; in Step 2, add them to the hot oil with the garlic and ginger and cook, stirring almost constantly until everything softens and browns in places, 1 or 2 minutes.

SQUID AND CABBAGE IN LETTUCE CUPS Substitute chopped squid for the chicken and 1 pound napa cabbage for the mushrooms and asparagus. In Step 2, it will only take 1 or 2 minutes to cook the squid through before adding the garlic and ginger.

PORK AND BEAN SPROUTS IN LETTUCE CUPS Swap ground pork for the chicken and 3 cups bean sprouts for the mushrooms and asparagus.

MORE IDEAS

Just before removing the chicken from the pan in Step 2, stir in 1 tablespoon curry powder or five-spice powder. • Add ½ cup coconut milk along with soy sauce. • Use fish sauce instead of soy sauce. • Substitute virtually any vegetable for those listed. In Step 4, add the ones that take the longest to soften to the pan first. • Try chopping up other meats, like trimmed pork shoulder, beef sirloin, or lamb leg, instead of the chicken. • Or try chopped peeled shrimp or scallops. Either will take half as long as the chicken to cook.

¼ cup mayonnaise (or Vegannaise; see page 242)

2 tablespoons fresh lime juice, or more to taste

2 tablespoons sriracha or other hot sauce, or to taste

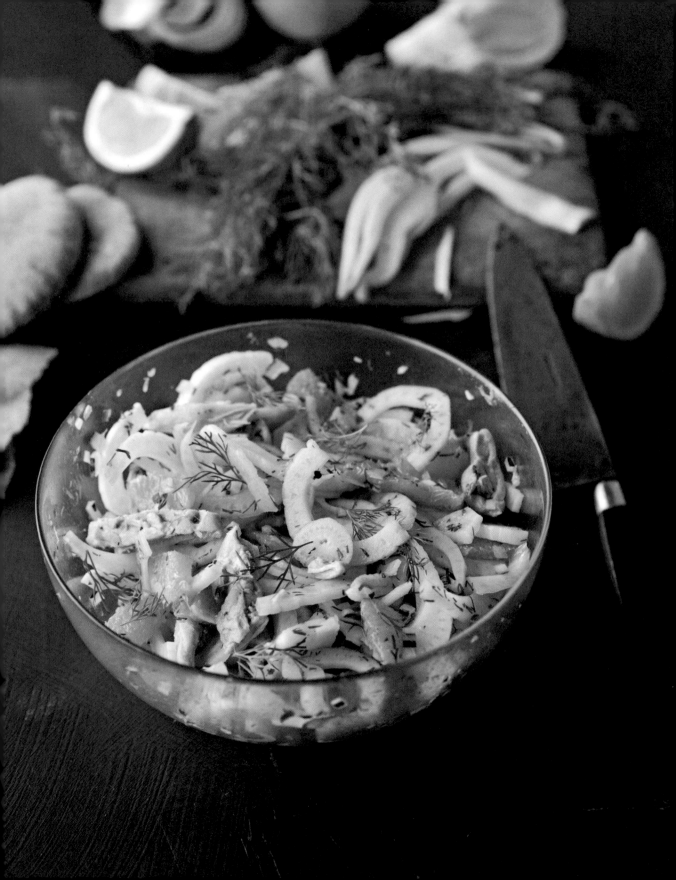

CHICKEN WITH FENNEL SALAD

MAKES 4 servings **TIME** 20 to 30 minutes

Quick, vibrant, and infinitely variable, this will join your repertoire of go-to weeknight dinners. Serve it with a whole-grain pita or other flat bread, or even tortillas. It's also good with plain rice or any other grain, or served on a bed of crisp greens.

1 fennel bulb, halved and thinly sliced

3 oranges, peeled, seeded if necessary, and chopped

1 small red onion, chopped

3 tablespoons olive oil

2 tablespoons chopped fresh dill, or 1 teaspoon dried

1 pound boneless chicken breasts, thighs, or tenders

1 teaspoon salt

½ teaspoon pepper

1 Prepare a grill or turn on the broiler; put the rack 4 inches from the heat source. Combine the fennel, oranges, onion, 2 tablespoons olive oil, the dill, and half the salt and pepper in a medium bowl. Let marinate, stirring once or twice while you cook the chicken.

2 Rub or brush the chicken with the remaining 1 tablespoon oil and sprinkle with the remaining ½ teaspoon salt and ¼ teaspoon pepper. When the grill or broiler is hot, put the chicken pieces directly on the grates or on a rimmed baking sheet under the broiler and cook, turning once, until browned and just cooked through, 3 to 5 minutes per side for breasts. (Figure 1 minute less per side for tenders and up to 5 minutes more per side for thighs.)

3 Taste and adjust the seasoning on the salad, and slice the chicken pieces as you like. Serve the chicken on top of a big scoop of the salad (or just toss everything all together).

VARIATIONS

CHICKEN CUTLETS WITH CELERY AND WATERMELON SALAD Only the salad changes. Use the center of the celery, including the leaves, instead of the fennel—you want about 2 cups chopped. Substitute 4 cups diced watermelon for the oranges and ¼ cup fresh mint for the dill. Cook the chicken as in the original recipe.

PORK MEDALLIONS WITH FENNEL AND APPLE SALAD Perfect with the season's first apples. Swap 1 pound pork tenderloin for the chicken; cut it crosswise into ¾-inch slices. Keep the fennel but try chopped apples instead of the oranges. Add 2 tablespoons lemon juice to the salad in Step 1.

MORE IDEAS

Other vegetables to try include radishes, kohlrabi, sunchokes, celery root, or carrots. • Other fruits to try are grapefruit, peaches, nectarines, plums, blackberries or strawberries, mango, papaya, pineapple, pears, figs, or any small citrus, like clementines or tangerines. If the fruit isn't very juicy, add some lemon or lime juice. • I often like to turn things upside down and make the bed-of-something into the topping. Try putting the meat on the plate first and spooning the salad on top. You might really like it.

GINGERED RICE WITH CHICKEN

MAKES 4 servings   TIME About 45 minutes, plus a little time to rest

Combine fried rice ingredients with a pilaf technique and you get an easy one-dish meal with a lot of flexibility. And a mix of silky and crisp vegetables, tender braised chicken, and rice with just the right bite. Once you put the lid on the pot, you're virtually home free, with plenty of time to make a salad or a dessert—or relax—while the rice steams.

1½ pounds bok choy

2 tablespoons vegetable oil

4 bone-in chicken thighs, skin removed

1 teaspoon salt

½ teaspoon pepper

1 large onion, chopped

2 tablespoons minced ginger

1½ cups brown rice, preferably basmati

2½ cups chicken or vegetable stock (see page 246), or water

1 cup fresh or frozen peas

1 Cut the bok choy leaves from the stalks and chop everything, keeping the leaves and stems separated. Put 1 tablespoon oil in a large skillet over medium heat. Add the chicken, sprinkle with half the salt and pepper, and cook undisturbed until the pieces brown and release easily from the pan, 3 to 5 minutes. Turn and brown on the other side, another 3 to 5 minutes. Remove the chicken from the pan and add the remaining 1 tablespoon oil.

2 Raise the heat to medium-high and add the onion and ginger. Cook, stirring, until the vegetables soften, 3 to 5 minutes. Add the rice all at once, turn the heat down to medium, and stir until the rice is glossy, completely coated with oil, and starting to color lightly, 3 to 5 minutes. Sprinkle with the remaining ½ teaspoon salt and ¼ teaspoon pepper, then add the stock all at once and bring to a boil, stirring once or twice.

3 Stir in the white parts of the bok choy, adjust the heat so the mixture bubbles gently, then nestle the chicken pieces on top and cover the pot. Cook without stirring until the rice is almost tender and the water is absorbed, 30 to 40 minutes.

4 When the rice is ready, remove the chicken and stir in the bok choy leaves and the peas with a fork. Turn the heat to the absolute minimum (if you have an electric stove, turn the heat off and let the pan sit on the burner) and let the pilaf rest for another 10 to 15 minutes. Taste and adjust the seasoning, fluff again, and serve the chicken on a bed of the rice.

RED OR GREEN RICE PILAF WITH CHICKEN Better known as *arroz rojo o verde con pollo*. Instead of ginger, use garlic; reduce the stock to 1¾ cups. Just before you add the stock, for *arroz rojo*, add about 1 cup chopped tomato; for *arroz verde*, add 1 cup chopped tomatillos. (In either case, canned is fine; don't bother to drain.) Substitute carrots for the bok choy. Garnish with cilantro and a squeeze of lemon or lime.

CHICKEN PILAF WITH OLIVES AND PINE NUTS Use olive oil instead of vegetable oil, and garlic instead of ginger. When you season the rice, add ½ teaspoon grated nutmeg. Substitute escarole for the bok choy, and ½ cup each chopped black olives and pine nuts for the peas.

KIMCHI CHICKEN RICE I love this. Substitute sesame oil for 1 tablespoon of the vegetable oil and use it instead of the second tablespoon oil at the end of Step 1. Skip the peas. Don't salt the rice in Step 2. When you add the bok choy leaves in Step 4, stir in 1 cup chopped kimchi. Pass soy sauce at the table.

MORE IDEAS

Change the greens: Chinese broccoli, chard, collards, or kale are all good here. • Add some heat: Toss in a couple (or more) of dried red chiles to the rice along with the salt and pepper. Or add chopped fresh chiles along with the bok choy leaves.

JERK CHICKEN BURGERS

MAKES 4 servings   **TIME** About 45 minutes

Jerk, as you probably know, is a Jamaican spice blend most often used as a rub or marinade for grilled chicken or pork. But it also works perfectly as a burger seasoning. And when you fold carrots and corn into the patty, and serve the whole thing on a crunchy and tangy cole slaw, you have a vegetable-driven one-plate meal that's anything but the same old thing.

3 tablespoons olive oil

2 tablespoons fresh lime juice

4 teaspoons minced garlic

1 teaspoon salt

½ teaspoon pepper

1 pound napa, savoy, or green cabbage, quartered and thinly sliced

1 large red or yellow bell pepper, thinly sliced

1 small red onion, halved and thinly sliced

1 pound ground chicken

1 carrot, grated

½ cup corn kernels, fresh or frozen

2 tablespoons jerk seasoning

¼ cup chopped fresh cilantro

1   Prepare a grill or turn on the broiler; put the rack 4 inches from the heat source. Put the olive oil in a large bowl with the lime juice, 2 teaspoons minced garlic, ½ teaspoon salt, and the pepper. Whisk until combined. Add the cabbage, bell pepper, and onion, and toss until the vegetables are coated in the dressing. Refrigerate the slaw for at least 10 minutes or up to several hours.

2   Combine the chicken, carrot, and corn with the jerk seasoning and the remaining 2 teaspoons garlic and ½ teaspoon salt. Handling the mixture as little as possible, shape the meat into four large or eight small burgers. (You can make them up to several hours ahead of cooking. Cover tightly and refrigerate; bring to room temperature before continuing.)

3   Put the burgers on the hot grill or on a rimmed baking sheet under the broiler, and cook undisturbed until they release from the grill grates easily (or if broiling, when they begin to brown on top), 5 to 7 minutes. Turn and cook the other side the same way. Check for doneness by taking a peek with a sharp knife. (When the burgers are ready the interior will no longer be pink and the juices will run clear.)

4   Stir the cilantro into the slaw, taste and adjust the seasoning, and serve the burgers right away, with the slaw on top.

VARIATION

CHICKEN BURGERS WITH VIETNAMESE FLAVORS Use peanut oil instead of olive oil in the slaw and add 1 or 2 minced small fresh red chiles (like Thai). Instead of jerk seasoning, use five-spice powder in the burgers and add 1 tablespoon fish sauce to the mixture instead of the remaining salt. Try substituting fresh mint or Thai basil in the slaw for the cilantro.

MORE IDEAS

Ground pork is a natural alternative in the burgers. Beef is great too. • If you're feeling more ambitious, pulse 1 pound peeled shrimp in a food processor and try that instead of the chicken in the burgers. • Eat the burger and slaw on a toasted bun (whole-grain or otherwise).

CHICKEN VEGETABLE TAGINE

MAKES 4 servings   TIME About 1 hour

Don't let the number of ingredients here scare you; this is an easy stew to make, and in fact you can substitute any number of them and you'll still be fine. The brightness of the cooked lemon is essential, however.

3 tablespoons vegetable oil

4 bone-in chicken drum-sticks (about 1½ pounds)

1 teaspoon salt

½ teaspoon pepper

1 pound eggplant, unpeeled, cubed

1 large onion, chopped

1 red bell pepper, chopped

1 tablespoon minced garlic

1 tablespoon minced ginger

1 teaspoon ground coriander

2 teaspoons ground cumin

1 teaspoon ground cinnamon

½ vanilla bean, or 1 teaspoon vanilla extract

4 cups chopped tomatoes (canned are fine; include their juice)

2 cups chicken or vegetable stock (see page 246), or water

1 lemon, scrubbed and chopped

4 cups cooked whole wheat couscous (page 230)

½ cup chopped fresh parsley, for garnish

1   Put 2 tablespoons oil in a large pot over medium-high heat. When it's hot, add the chicken and cook, turning and rotating the pieces as necessary, and sprinkling with the salt and pepper, until the drumsticks are well browned on all sides, 10 to 15 minutes. Transfer the chicken to a large bowl.

2   Turn the heat down to medium and add the eggplant. Cook, stirring occasionally, until it softens and browns in places, 15 to 20 minutes; add water, a little at a time as the eggplant cooks to keep it from sticking to the pan and burning. Transfer the eggplant to the bowl with the chicken.

3   Add the remaining 1 tablespoon oil to the pan along with the onion, bell pepper, garlic, and ginger and cook, stirring frequently until the vegetables soften, 3 to 5 minutes. Add the coriander, cumin, cinnamon, and the vanilla bean, if you're using it (if you're using extract, wait). Cook, stirring, until fragrant, no more than 1 minute.

4   Pour in the tomatoes and stock, and bring to a boil, scraping the bottom of the pot to loosen any browned bits. Return the chicken and eggplant to the pan; if you're using extract, add it now. Add the lemon; when the stew returns to a boil, lower the heat so it bubbles gently but steadily, and cover. Cook, stirring once or twice, until the chicken is almost falling off the bone and the vegetables are quite tender, 20 to 30 minutes. Taste and adjust the seasoning. Spoon the tagine over the couscous, garnish with parsley, and serve.

VARIATION

VEGETABLE AND CHICKPEA TAGINE   Swap 3 cups cooked or canned chickpeas (or mature fava beans, or frozen green fava or lima beans) for the chicken. Add along with the lemon in Step 4. Use vegetable stock instead of chicken stock if you want to make it vegan.

MORE IDEAS

Try this with cubed lamb shoulder or beef chuck. • Up the vegetables by stirring kale into the pot when you add the couscous. • Add up to ½ cup raisins or dried apricots along with (or instead of) the chopped lemon. • Top this dish with toasted pine nuts or almonds for some crunch.

AFRICAN-STYLE CHICKEN STEW

MAKES 4 servings   **TIME** 45 minutes

My spin on the peanut soups of West Africa has evolved over the years. These days I'm making a less soupy version and loading it up with collards. Try it: It's the best use of peanut butter I know (aside from on crackers, of course).

2 tablespoons vegetable oil

1 pound skinless, boneless chicken thighs, cut into 1½-inch chunks

1 teaspoon salt

½ teaspoon pepper

1 onion, halved and thinly sliced

1 tablespoon minced garlic

1 tablespoon minced ginger

Pinch cayenne (optional)

2 cups chicken or vegetable stock (page 246), or water

4 cups chopped tomatoes (canned are fine; include their juice)

½ pound sweet potatoes or yams, peeled and chopped

1 pound collards or kale, chopped

¼ cup chunky peanut butter

¼ cup chopped roasted peanuts, for garnish

1   Put the oil in a large pot over medium-high heat. When it's hot, add the chicken, sprinkle with half the salt and pepper, and cook, stirring occasionally and adjusting the heat so they sizzle without burning, until the pieces are browned all over, 5 to 10 minutes. Add the onion, garlic, ginger, remaining ½ teaspoon salt and ¼ teaspoon pepper, and the cayenne if you're using it. Cook, stirring occasionally, until the vegetables are soft, 3 to 5 minutes.

2   Add the stock, tomatoes, and sweet potatoes; bring to a boil; then turn the heat down so that the stew bubbles gently but steadily. Cover the pot and cook, stirring occasionally, until the potatoes are just getting tender, 8 to 12 minutes.

3   Add the collards and peanut butter and stir. Cover again and cook until the greens are tender, 15 to 20 minutes. Taste, adjust the seasoning, and serve, garnished with peanuts.

VARIATIONS

AFRICAN PEANUT SOUP WITH RICE Thicker, especially if you let the rice cook until the kernels burst. Substitute ½ cup long-grain brown rice for the sweet potatoes and add an extra cup of stock. In Step 2, let the rice cook until it's almost fully tender before proceeding, 25 to 30 minutes.

BEEF STEW WITH PISTACHIOS, BEETS, AND GREENS Perfect for whenever you can get your hands on lots of beet greens, but any green will do. Substitute beef sirloin for the chicken, beets for the sweet potatoes, the beet greens for the collards, and pistachios for the peanuts.

MORE IDEAS

Cashews are always a good substitute for peanuts. So are sesame, sunflower, and pumpkin seeds. • Instead of the sweet potatoes, try carrots, parsnips, celery root, or an interesting tropical tuber like taro or boniato. • If you like chiles, try using minced fresh red chiles (like serrano or Thai bird) instead of the cayenne. • Ground chicken—or any ground meat, for that matter—gives this a pleasantly grainy texture. • You might consider cutting the vegetables smaller. Or not.

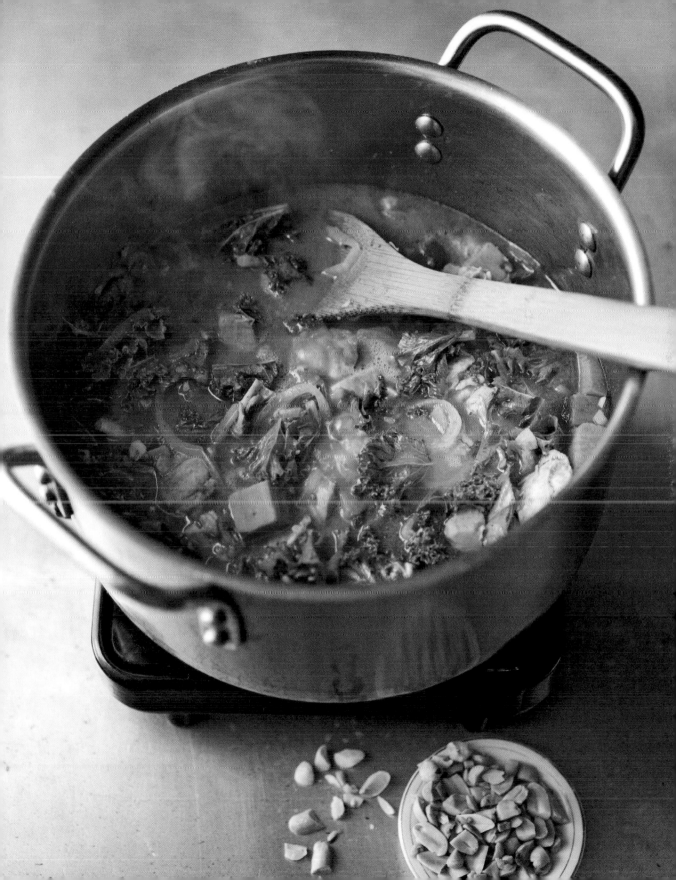

PROVENÇAL CHICKEN STEW

MAKES 4 servings   TIME 45 minutes

I can eat almost anything that's topped with olive-oil fried breadcrumbs, especially this combination inspired by the iconic dishes of southern France. It may seem like a lot of spinach, but it cooks down to a fraction of its volume—and is really tender and delicious.

1 cup cooked or canned chickpeas (see page 232)

4 tablespoons olive oil

1 cup whole wheat breadcrumbs (see page 251)

1 teaspoon salt

½ teaspoon pepper

1 pound boneless chicken breasts

1 tablespoon minced garlic

2 pounds spinach

2 cups chicken or vegetable stock (see page 246)

Pinch red chile flakes (optional)

1   Drain the chickpeas. If you made them yourself, reserve the cooking liquid; if they're canned, discard it and rinse the chickpeas. Put 2 table-spoons oil in a large skillet over medium heat. When it's hot, add the breadcrumbs, sprinkle with ¼ teaspoon each of the salt and pepper, and cook, stirring frequently until they're crisp and toasted, 3 to 5 minutes. Remove them from the pan.

2   Add the remaining 2 tablespoons oil to the skillet and turn the heat to medium-high. When it's hot, add the chicken, sprinkle with ½ teaspoon of the remaining salt, and cook until the breasts are well browned and release easily from the pan, 3 to 5 minutes. Turn and cook on the other side the same way. Remove them from the pan.

3   Add the garlic to the drippings in the pan and turn the heat back down to medium. Stir, then start adding the spinach a handful at a time; keep stirring until all the spinach fits in the pan and starts to release its water; sprinkle with the remaining ¼ teaspoon salt and pepper. Then add the stock, the chickpeas, and the red chile flakes if you're using them. Adjust the heat so the mixture bubbles gently but steadily, then return the chicken to the pan. Cover and cook just long enough for the chicken to cook through, 1 or 2 minutes more.

4   Taste the spinach and adjust the seasoning. Slice the chicken cross-wise against the grain to any thickness you like. Divide the spinach and broth among bowls, put some chicken on top, sprinkle the breadcrumbs over all, and serve.

VARIATION

TUSCAN CHICKEN STEW   The title here says it all: Swap sliced zucchini (or summer squash) for the spinach and cannellini beans for the chickpeas. In Step 3, you'll need to cook the vegetables longer before returning the chicken to the pot; figure 5 to 10 minutes more.

MORE IDEAS

If you've got homemade chickpeas (and their precious cooking liquid, see page 232), then substitute the cooked liquid for some or all of the stock.
• Season the breadcrumbs with chopped fresh parsley or basil.

GINGERY WINTER STEW

MAKES **4 servings**   TIME **At least 1 hour, largely unattended**

Any hard winter squash—butternut, pumpkin, acorn—will work perfectly in this satisfying and attractive cold-weather braise. If you see kabocha, grab it; it's got unique flesh, which is silky, meaty, and pleasantly tender all at the same time. And it's the kind of dish that's easy to change with the season (see the first variation). A scoop of brown rice is the perfect accompaniment here all year round.

2 tablespoons olive oil

1 pounds pork shoulder, cut into 1½-inch chunks

½ teaspoon salt

½ teaspoon pepper

1 large onion, chopped

2 apples, peeled and chopped

¼ cup minced ginger

2 cups vegetable or chicken stock (see page 246), or water, plus more as needed

¼ cup soy sauce

2 tablespoons lemon juice

2 pounds any winter squash, cut into 1-inch chunks

1 Put the oil in a large pot over medium-high heat. When it's hot, add the pork, sprinkle with the salt and pepper, and cook, turning the pieces as they release easily from the pan, until they're well browned on all sides, 10 to 15 minutes. If necessary work in two batches to avoid crowding. As the meat finishes cooking, remove it from the pot.

2 Add the onion, apples, and ginger to the pot and cook until they begin to soften, 3 to 5 minutes. Add the stock, soy sauce, and lemon juice and bring to a boil, stirring to scrape up any brown bits from the bottom of the pot. Add the browned pork and adjust the heat so the mixture bubbles gently but steadily and cover.

3 After 30 minutes, begin to check the meat every 15 minutes. When the meat is tender enough to fall easily from a fork, stir in the squash. Cook, stirring occasionally and adding enough more stock to keep it from sticking, until the squash is tender but not mushy, 10 to 15 minutes. Taste and adjust the seasoning and serve.

VARIATIONS

GINGERY SUMMER STEW Totally different—and lighter, to mirror the season. If you'd like, use beef chuck instead of the pork. Substitute tomatoes for the apples and zucchini for the winter squash. Add ¼ cup chopped fresh mint or ½ cup chopped fresh basil just before serving.

GARLICKY WINTER OR SUMMER STEW Use garlic instead of ginger for a different kind of heat.

MORE IDEAS

Go green: Substitute chopped chard or kale for some or all of the squash. • Instead of soy sauce, use half the amount of fish sauce. Try lime instead of lemon juice. • Use a different meat. This would also be fantastic with either beef chuck or lamb shoulder or shank. • Try pears instead of apples.

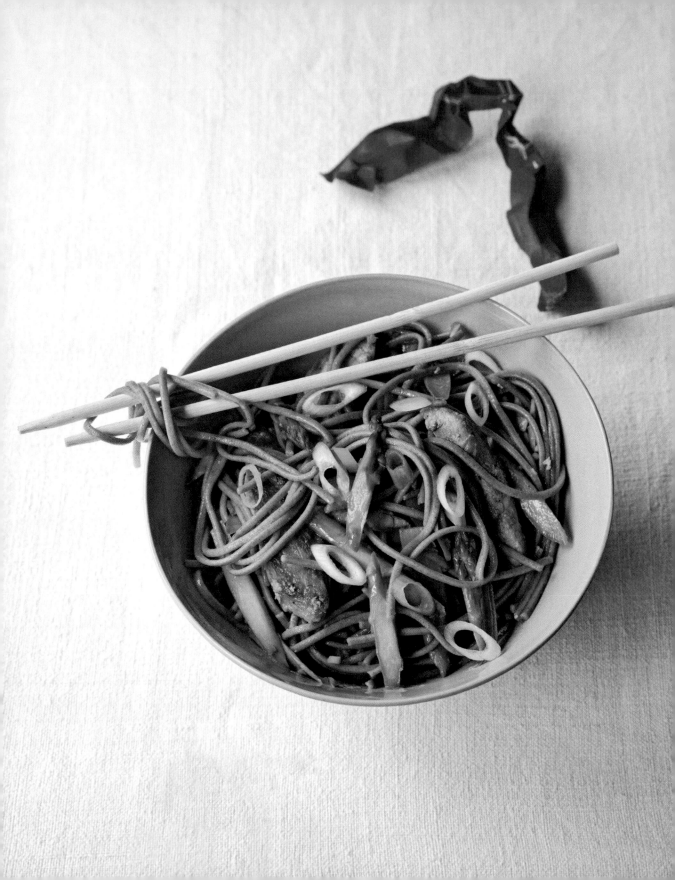

PORK, ASPARAGUS, AND SOBA

MAKES 4 servings   TIME About 30 minutes

A favorite of mine. Asparagus is built for this combination dry-and-wet cooking method, since a single stalk runs the gamut of different textures, from the crispest stalk ends to the tender tips. Peel the stalks (which I take the time to do if they're more than pencil-thin) or not—it's your call. The best way to cut them is on the bias to maximize the surface area. (They look nice that way too.)

1½ teaspoons salt

2 tablespoons vegetable oil

1 pound pork shoulder, cut into thin strips

½ teaspoon pepper

1 tablespoon minced garlic

1 tablespoon minced ginger

1 small dried hot red chile (like Thai), or pinch of red chile flakes, or more to taste

8 ounces soba noodles

1 tablespoon sesame oil

1½ pounds asparagus (thick ends peeled if you like), thinly cut on an angle

1 tablespoon soy sauce, or to taste

2 scallions, sliced, for garnish

1   Bring a large pot of water to a boil and add 1 teaspoon salt. Put a large skillet over high heat. Add 1 tablespoon oil, swirl it around, and immediately add the pork and sprinkle it with the remaining ½ teaspoon salt and the pepper. Cook undisturbed until the pieces brown and release from the pan easily. Then add the garlic, ginger, and chile and stir frequently, until the meat is no longer pink and the vegetables soften, 3 to 5 minutes total. Remove the meat mixture from the pan and the pan from the heat.

2   Cook the noodles in the boiling water until tender but not mushy. Start checking them after 3 minutes. Drain the noodles, reserving about 1 cup of the cooking water, and toss the soba with the sesame oil.

3   Return the skillet to medium-high heat and add the asparagus along with ¼ cup water, stirring to scrape up any browned bits from the bottom of the pan. Cook until the asparagus is dry and beginning to brown, 5 to 10 minutes. Add a little more water if necessary to prevent them from burning.

4   Stir in the soy sauce, noodles, and a small splash of the noodle-cooking water; return the pork to the skillet. Cook, stirring and adding just enough water to keep everything from sticking, until the pork and noodles are hot, no more than 1 minute. Taste and adjust the seasoning, adding more soy sauce if necessary. Garnish with the scallions and serve hot or at room temperature.

(recipe continues)

BEEF, BROCCOLI, AND SOBA Swap thinly sliced beef sirloin (or, if you're feeling indulgent, rib-eye or strip steak) for the pork, and broccoli florets for the asparagus. (Or try cutting the florets into thin planks that look like the cross-sections of trees.)

SQUID, ASPARAGUS, AND RICE NOODLES Get a Vietnamese profile in a flash. Use sliced squid instead of pork; in Step 1, cook, stirring, until it's just opaque, 2 or 3 minutes. Skip the ginger; use rice vermicelli instead of soba (and soak it in boiling water for 3 to 5 minutes instead of boiling it); substitute fish sauce for the soy sauce; and garnish with chopped fresh Thai or other basil instead of the scallions. Serve with lime wedges.

MORE IDEAS

Other vegetables to try include carrots, bell peppers or mild chiles, celery, cauliflower, snow peas, or green beans. • Any protein will work here, even seafood; just adjust the cooking time in Step 1 so quick-to-cook foods like shrimp don't get overdone and tough. • Add a little acidity, especially if you're serving this dish at room temperature. A tablespoon of rice vinegar or lemon or lime juice should do the trick.

CRISP PORK ON GREEN PAPAYA SALAD

MAKES 4 servings   **TIME** About 45 minutes

A traditional Thai salad, served everywhere from food carts to fine restaurants. Here, I top the papaya—which can be found at Asian grocery stores and many supermarkets—with pork marinated in *nam pla prik*, or fresh chili-fish sauce. See the ideas that follow for some simple substitutions.

1 pound boneless pork loin chops

5 tablespoons fresh lime juice

¼ cup fish sauce

1 tablespoon minced garlic

3 fresh chiles (more or less), preferably Thai, seeded and minced

2 teaspoons sugar, preferably turbinado

1 large green, unripe papaya, peeled and seeded

1 shallot, minced

2 or 3 long beans, or 12 or so green beans, cut into ½-inch lengths

1 large tomato, chopped

2 tablespoons vegetable oil

½ teaspoon salt

½ teaspoon pepper

2 tablespoons chopped dry-roasted peanuts

½ cup chopped fresh cilantro, for garnish

1 Put the pork in the freezer while you get the other ingredients ready. Whisk together the lime juice, fish sauce, garlic, some of the chile, and the sugar in a large bowl. Transfer one-third of the dressing to a medium bowl and keep it handy.

2 Cut the papaya into fine shreds either by hand with a sharp knife, on a mandoline, or with the julienne disk of a food processor. You should have about 4 cups. Add the papaya along with the shallot, beans, and tomato to the bowl; toss a few times, and refrigerate.

3 Slice the pork against the grain as thin as possible. Put the oil in a large skillet over high heat. When it's hot, add the pork, sprinkle with the salt and pepper, and cook undisturbed until it sizzles, browns around the edges, and releases easily from the pan, 1 or 2 minutes. Cook and stir until the meat loses most—but not all—of its pink. Transfer the meat to the bowl with the reserved dressing and stir.

4 Return the skillet to medium heat, stir in ½ cup water, and cook, stirring and scraping up any browned bits from the bottom of the pan. Let the mixture bubble away until only a syrup remains; pour it into the bowl with the pork and stir. Taste and adjust the seasoning of both the salad and the pork. Serve the marinated meat on top of the papaya salad, topped with the peanuts and garnished with the cilantro.

VARIATION

SEARED BEEF ON MANGO-CUCUMBER SALAD Substitute beef sirloin for the pork and ginger for the garlic. Instead of the papaya, peel, seed, and thinly slice 2 mangos and 1 large cucumber.

MORE IDEAS

Instead of the papaya, try Granny Smith apples, cucumber, napa cabbage, or kohlrabi. (Trim, peel, and core them as you normally do, but be sure to seed the cucumber for best results.) • Instead of the green beans, try thinly sliced snow peas or shiitake mushrooms, or bean sprouts.

PORK CHOP PAN ROAST

MAKES 4 servings   **TIME** 1 hour and 30 minutes, largely unattended

Roasting lots of colorful root vegetables with dried fruit, nuts, and just enough pork makes for a gorgeous dish that's hearty without being heavy. Imagine a hash that's not quite stirred together so you get the same kind of big flavor meld, only with perfectly cooked meat and vegetables in every bite. (And, if you actually would prefer hash, there's a variation for that as well.)

2 tablespoons minced garlic

1 tablespoon chopped fresh sage, or 1 teaspoon dried sage

1 teaspoon salt

½ teaspoon pepper

2 pounds beets, cut into ½-inch chunks

4 large carrots, cut into ½-inch chunks

1 large red onion, cut into ½-inch chunks

3 tablespoons olive oil

2 thick bone-in pork loin chops (1½ pounds total)

¼ cup golden raisins

¼ cup chopped dates

¼ cup chopped pistachios or almonds

1   Heat the oven to 425°F. Mix the garlic, sage, salt, and pepper in a small bowl. Put the beets, carrots, and onion in a large roasting pan and toss them with the olive oil and about 1 teaspoon of the garlic-sage mixture. Transfer the pan to the oven and cook undisturbed until the vegetables begin to soften, 5 to 10 minutes.

2   Meanwhile, make shallow slits all over the pork with a small, sharp knife. Insert most of the remaining garlic-sage mixture into the slits and spread the rest all over the outsides. Remove the vegetables from the oven and stir. Nestle the chops into the pan so that they touch the bottom and the vegetables surround them; return the pan to the oven.

3   Roast until the bottoms of the chops are browned and they release easily from the pan, 10 to 15 minutes. Turn them, stir the vegetables, and reposition the meat. Cook undisturbed until the vegetables are barely tender and just starting to brown, but the meat is still a little more rare than you ultimately want it, 5 to 10 minutes more. Remove the chops from the pan, stir the vegetables and spread them around, and return them to the oven while the meat rests.

4   Let the chops sit for at least 5 minutes and up to 10 minutes. When the vegetables are fully tender and the meat is ready, add the fruit and nuts to the vegetables and stir. Taste and adjust the seasoning. To serve, first slice the meat off the bones in one piece (save the bones for making soup), then cut the pork into thick slices and fan them out on top of the vegetables.

PORK CHOP HASH Made easier since it's simply roasted. Get the vegetables started as described in Step 1. Instead of slitting and seasoning the meat in Step 2, cut the meat off the bone and into 1-inch chunks; toss the pieces with the remaining sage mixture, then add the meat to the vegetables. Continue to roast, stirring occasionally, until the vegetables are tender, the pork is crisp, and everything is well browned, 20 to 30 minutes total.

SLICED PORK WITH PUREED VEGETABLES After you remove the meat from the pan in Step 4, transfer the vegetables to a blender. Add 1 cup chicken or vegetable stock (or water) to the pan and set it over two burners turned to medium-high heat. Cook, stirring constantly and scraping up any browned bits, until the liquid boils, then transfer it to the blender. Puree the vegetables until smooth and use that as the base for the sliced pork.

MORE IDEAS

You can use thyme, rosemary, oregano, or marjoram instead of the sage.
• Instead of the beets and carrots, try parsnips, turnips, sweet potatoes, celery root, or rutabagas.

HAM HASH WITH GREENS

MAKES 4 servings   **TIME** About 1 hour

Consider this two-pan roasting technique a master recipe that works for all sorts of vegetable-and-meat combinations. Because the results reheat well—and are quite fine at room temperature—you can make the dish in advance to serve a group or to have tasty leftovers. All you might need on the side is a cup of soup.

1½ pounds sweet potatoes, peeled and cut into 1-inch chunks

2 tablespoons olive oil

1 teaspoon salt

½ teaspoon pepper

1½ pounds collards, stems and ribs removed; leaves chopped

1 teaspoon minced garlic

2 tablespoons red wine vinegar

1 onion, chopped

12 ounces cooked ham, cut into ½-inch chunks

1   Heat the oven to 400°F and adjust the racks so there is some room between them. Put the sweet potatoes on a large rimmed baking sheet, drizzle with 1 tablespoon oil and sprinkle with ½ teaspoon salt and pepper, and toss to coat. Transfer the pan to the oven and roast undisturbed for 20 minutes, then check. If the potatoes release easily from the pan, loosen and toss them with a spatula. If not, wait until they do, checking every 5 minutes or so.

2   Meanwhile, on another large rimmed baking sheet, drizzle collards with the remaining tablespoon oil and ½ teaspoon salt. Rub the leaves together with your hands to evenly distribute the seasoning and bruise them a bit. Add the garlic and vinegar, toss, and spread out in the pan.

3   Add the onion and ham to the sweet potatoes, toss to combine, and continue roasting. Put the pan with the collards in the oven above the potatoes. Cook, stirring the contents of both pans occasionally, until the vegetables are tender but the greens are not overly crisp, 15 to 20 minutes. Transfer all vegetables, ham, and collards to a large bowl and cover with a sheet of foil to steam for 5 minutes. Taste and adjust the seasoning and serve.

VARIATIONS

PROSCIUTTO HASH   Talk about decadent, and a little more subtle than ham. Use bits of prosciutto instead of ham and lacinato kale instead of collards. A sprinkle of Parmesan cheese at the end wouldn't hurt.

SAUSAGE HASH   A hearty alternative. Use chopped hot or sweet Italian sausage instead of the ham and add it in Step 1 when you start the potatoes. Substitute escarole for the collards. Add a pinch of red chile flakes if you like.

MORE IDEAS

In summer, try cherry tomatoes instead of the collard greens. Let them roast just long enough to wrinkle a bit, 5 or 10 minutes tops. • You can always take the traditional route and use regular potatoes instead of sweet potatoes. • Your choice: waxy (like red-skinned or fingerlings), starchy (like russets), or in between (like Yukon Gold).

SWEET POTATO SHEPHERD'S PIE

MAKES 4 servings   TIME 1 hour, partially unattended

A British pub favorite, this quintessential casserole is usually made by smothering leftover meat and gravy with mashed potatoes before baking. But there are as many renditions as there are cooks.

1½ pounds sweet potatoes, peeled and cut into chunks

2 teaspoons salt

3 tablespoons olive oil

12 ounces ground beef or lamb

1 onion, chopped

1 carrot, chopped

½ head green cabbage (about 1 pound), chopped

½ teaspoon pepper

1 tablespoon tomato paste

1 tablespoon chopped fresh thyme, or 1 teaspoon dried

1 cup fresh or frozen peas

½ cup white beans

1½ cups beef or chicken stock (see page 246), or water

1 Heat the oven to 400°F. Put the sweet potatoes in a large pot with enough water to cover by 2 inches and 1 teaspoon salt. Bring to a boil, lower the heat so the water bubbles steadily, and cook, stirring once or twice, until they're tender, 15 to 20 minutes. Drain the potatoes thoroughly, and mash them with 1 tablespoon olive oil and ¼ teaspoon salt until smooth.

2 Meanwhile, put 1 tablespoon oil in a 10- or 12-inch ovenproof skillet over medium-high heat. Add the meat and cook, stirring frequently and breaking it up, until it browns and crisps in places, 3 to 5 minutes. Transfer it to a plate.

3 Put the remaining 1 tablespoon oil in the pan and return it to medium heat. Add the onion, carrot, and cabbage; sprinkle with the remaining 1¾ teaspoons salt and the pepper; and cook, stirring occasionally until the vegetables soften, 5 to 10 minutes. Add the tomato paste, thyme, and peas along with the browned meat; stir until combined, adjusting the heat so the mixture doesn't burn. Mash the beans and stock together with a fork and add them to the pan, stirring again to combine and thicken. Taste and adjust the seasoning.

4 Spread the sweet potatoes over the meat mixture, and bake until the filling is bubbly and the edges begin to brown, 25 to 35 minutes. Serve hot.

VARIATIONS

TURKEY SHEPHERD'S PIE I'm a fan of using leftover turkey to make shepherd's pie, especially after Thanksgiving. Omit the ground beef or lamb and skip Step 2. When the vegetables are soft in Step 3, stir in 3 cups chopped cooked turkey before adding the tomato paste.

PORK PIE Red cabbage and onion are nice here. Use ground pork for the meat and sage instead of thyme.

VEGAN SHEPHERD'S PIE Use 2 pounds sliced button or cremini mushrooms instead of the meat. Cook them as directed in Step 2, only longer—until they release their water and then become dry and brown, 10 to 15 minutes. Use vegetable stock instead of beef stock.

PARSNIP-TOPPED SHEPHERD'S PIE Substitute cooked and pureed parsnips for the sweet potatoes.

BÁNH MÌ MEATBALL SALAD

MAKES 4 servings   TIME 45 minutes

Here I turn a trendy—and traditional—Vietnamese sandwich into a meal-size salad. All the components are here: crisp greens, pickled vegetables, spicy meatballs, and crusty bread (which appears here as croutons). And since you can mix and roll the meatballs and pickle the vegetables in advance, this salad has party written all over it.

⅓ cup rice vinegar

1 teaspoon maple syrup or other sweetener

1 teaspoon salt

2 carrots, cut into thin strips or grated

½ large daikon, cut into thin strips or grated

3 or 4 large shallots, or 1 medium red onion, halved and thinly sliced

One 8-ounce baguette, cut or torn into 1-inch pieces

3 tablespoons vegetable oil

1 pound ground beef

1 tablespoon minced garlic

¼ teaspoon red chile flakes, or to taste

½ teaspoon pepper

1 tablespoon fish sauce

1½ pounds romaine lettuce, torn into bite-size pieces (about 8 cups)

2 pints cherry tomatoes

1 large cucumber, peeled and seeded if necessary, chopped

½ cup chopped fresh cilantro or mint, for garnish

Lime wedges

1 Whisk the vinegar, syrup, and ½ teaspoon salt together in a medium bowl. Add the carrots, daikon, and shallots and toss gently. Refrigerate for at least 30 minutes; stir it every once in a while to distribute the brine. (You can refrigerate the pickles in an airtight container for up to several days.)

2 When you're ready to eat, heat the oven to 450°F. Put the bread on a rimmed baking sheet and bake, shaking the pan occasionally, until lightly toasted, 5 to 10 minutes. Remove the croutons from the baking sheet and drizzle with 1 tablespoon oil.

3 Combine the beef, garlic, red chile flakes, pepper, fish sauce, and ¼ teaspoon salt in a medium bowl. Gently shape the meat into 12 medium or 16 small meatballs, handling them as little as possible. (The meatballs can be shaped up to a day in advance, covered, and refrigerated.) Transfer the meatballs to the prepared pan and bake undisturbed until they're browned, 8 to 12 minutes. Let them cool a bit while you assemble the salad.

4 Put the lettuce, tomatoes, and cucumber in a large bowl with the pickled vegetables. Drizzle with the remaining 2 tablespoons oil, sprinkle with the remaining ¼ teaspoon salt, and toss. Add the croutons and toss again. Divide the salad among bowls, top with the meatballs, garnish with the herb, and serve with the lime wedges.

OPEN-FACE BÁNH MÌ SANDWICHES Like bruschetta with salad on top; very pretty. Slice the bread horizontally instead of making croutons. Everything else remains the same. When the meatballs are cool enough to handle, slice them in half. Put the bread on a plate, top first with the meatballs, then the salad.

BÁNH MÌ MEATBALL SALAD WITH SRIRACHA DRESSING This change goes for the main recipe and all the variations and ideas. Instead of dressing the salad with the oil before tossing in Step 4, stir 2 tablespoons mayonnaise (or Vegannaise, page 242) into the pickled vegetables and add sriracha to taste.

MORE IDEAS

Use ground turkey, pork, or chicken instead of the pork. • Season the meatballs with 2 tablespoons minced lemongrass or fresh Thai basil. • Avocado is a fantastic addition, though not entirely traditional. • If you've got leftovers handy, speed things up and try sliced roast or grilled beef or pork, or shredded chicken or turkey instead of the meatballs.

SCHEZUAN BEEF AND CELERY

MAKES 4 servings   **TIME** 30 minutes, plus time for freezing the meat

Once you master the rhythm of a stir-fry you open up a world of recipes. This one is a riff off the traditional dry-fried (and assertively seasoned!) Szechuan beef. It involves sweet bean paste (akin to miso, only stronger) and Schezuan peppercorns, which leave a tingly sensation and spicy flavor behind. You'll find these readily at any Asian market, but I've listed alternatives, as well as tamer options, among the variations. For a change from rice, serve this stir-fry with soba or brown rice noodles.

1 pound beef flank or sirloin steak

3 tablespoons vegetable oil

1 teaspoon salt

1 bunch scallions, white and green parts separated, both chopped

1 tablespoon minced ginger

1 tablespoon minced fresh hot chile (like jalapeño or Thai)

1 tablespoon sweet bean sauce or red or brown miso

1 teaspoon crushed Schezuan peppercorns or five-spice blend

½ teaspoon pepper

1 teaspoon maple syrup or other sweetener

1 large bunch celery, leaves and stalks separated, both chopped

1 If you have time, put the steak in the freezer for 10 or 20 minutes while you get the other ingredients ready. Slice the meat across the grain as thin as you can. Put a large, deep skillet over high heat. When it's hot, add 1 tablespoon oil, swirl it around, and add the beef. Sprinkle with ½ teaspoon salt and cook, stirring occasionally, until the beef browns all over, 3 to 5 minutes. Transfer to a plate.

2 Add the remaining 2 tablespoons oil to the skillet, swirl it around, then add the white parts of the scallions, the ginger, chile, sweet bean sauce, peppercorns, pepper, and the remaining ½ teaspoon salt. Cook and stir until fragrant, no more than 1 minute. Add the syrup and ½ cup water and stir until a sauce forms, just 30 seconds or so.

3 Add the celery stalks to the pan and cook, stirring occasionally, until they're brightly colored and the pan is almost dry, 1 or 2 minutes. Return the beef to the skillet along with the scallion greens and celery leaves. Stir to combine, taste and adjust the seasoning, and serve.

VARIATIONS

BEEF AND CELERY STIR-FRY WITH SOY SAUCE Skip the sweet bean sauce, Schezuan peppercorns, and chile. In Step 2, add 1 tablespoon minced garlic. When you add the water in Step 3, stir in 2 tablespoons soy sauce and the juice of 1 lemon.

SWEET-AND-SOUR BEEF AND CELERY STIR-FRY Sweet-and-Sour flavor with real ingredients. Follow the variation above, except instead of the lemon juice use 2 tablespoons rice vinegar. When you add the celery in Step 3, toss in 2 cups diced fresh pineapple.

MORE IDEAS

Add crunch: Toss in ½ cup chopped cashews just before serving. • Vary the protein: pork loin, boneless chicken thighs, lamb shoulder, or even sliced tofu are all fair game.

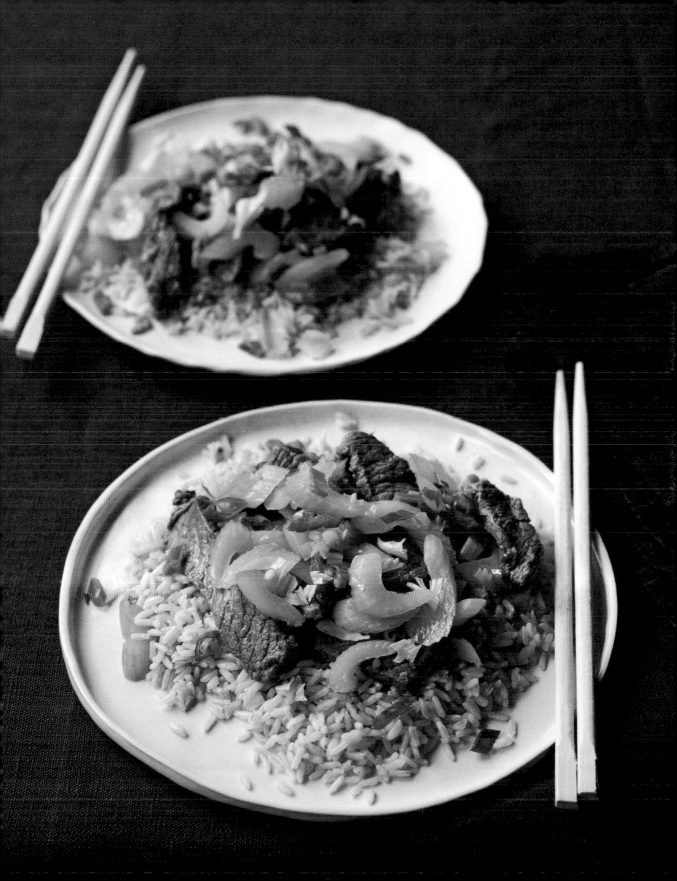

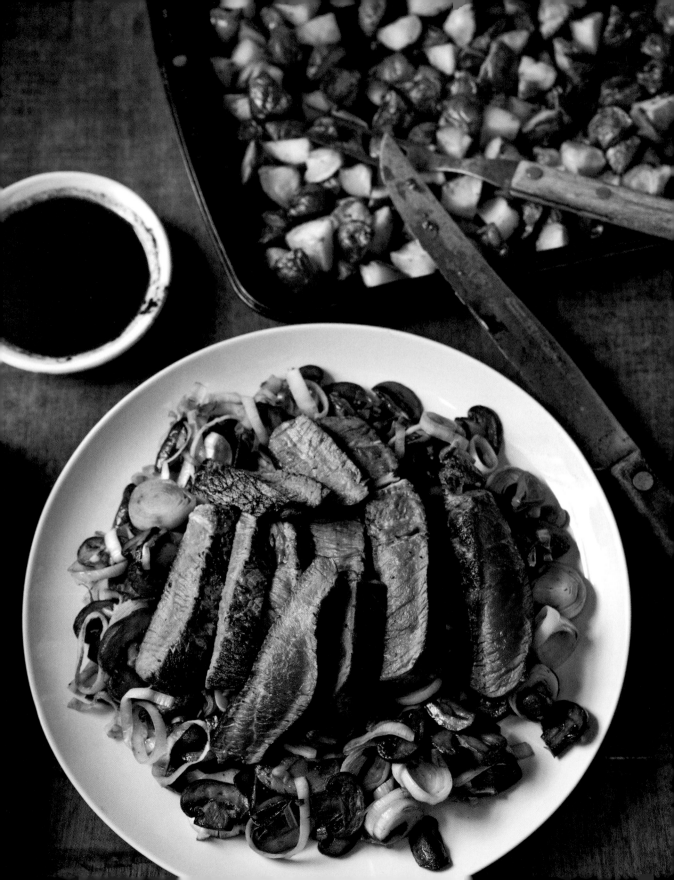

STEAK AU POIVRE WITH MUSHROOMS

MAKES 4 servings   TIME 45 minutes

Pan-cooked mushrooms can be irresistibly delicious, especially when paired with steak. The trick is to stir them just enough to prevent burning, but infrequently enough to let them caramelize a bit. (Same with the leeks, whose sweetness contributes mightily.)

3 tablespoons olive oil

2 pounds mushrooms (like button or cremini), sliced

1 teaspoon salt

2 leeks, rinsed well and sliced crosswise

1 tablespoon chopped fresh tarragon, or ½ teaspoon dried

1 pound beef sirloin, rib eye, strip, or other steak (about 1 inch thick)

1 tablespoon pepper

¾ cup red wine or water

1   Heat the oven to 200°F. Put 2 tablespoons oil in a large skillet over medium heat. Add the mushrooms, sprinkle with ½ teaspoon salt, and cook, stirring occasionally, until they release their water and the pan begins to dry out again, 10 to 15 minutes. Add the leeks and cook, stirring occasionally until they soften a bit, 2 or 3 minutes. Add the tarragon and stir until fragrant, 30 seconds or so, then transfer the mushrooms and leeks to an ovenproof dish; put in the oven.

2   Put the remaining 1 tablespoon oil in the skillet and let it get hot. Sprinkle the remaining ½ teaspoon salt and the pepper into the hot fat, and immediately put the steak (or steaks) on top. Cook undisturbed until the meat develops a brown crust on the bottom and releases easily, 3 to 5 minutes. Turn and cook until the other side browns a little too and the steak is still a little more rare than you like it—no more than a couple more minutes. (The best way to know for sure is to nick the steak with a sharp knife and peek inside.)

3   Transfer the steak to a cutting board and add the wine to the skillet. Cook, stirring to loosen any browned bits and let the liquid reduce to a little less than ½ cup. Cut the steak across the grain into ½-inch slices and put them on top of the mushrooms and leeks. Pour the pan juices over all and serve.

VARIATION

PEPPER STEAK WITH ASPARAGUS AND SHALLOTS Instead of the mushrooms, slice 1½ pounds asparagus on the bias into 1-inch pieces. Substitute 3 large shallots for the leeks; cut them crosswise into thin rings. In Step 1, cook the shallots in the hot oil to give them a 2- or 3-minute head start, then add the asparagus and go from there.

MORE IDEAS

Stir ½ pound fresh spinach into the mushroom and leek mixture just before they're ready to be put in the oven. • Swap Marsala wine, port, or sherry for the red wine. • For genuine steak au poivre, coarsely grind about 1 table-spoon peppercorns and press them into the meat. Then just add the salt to the hot oil in Step 2.

GRITS AND GRILLADES

MAKES 4 servings   TIME About 2 to 3 hours, mostly unattended

A traditional New Orleans dish, grits and grillades—the latter a French word of various meanings, all related to tasty and fatty pieces of meat. This therefore can be made with beef, pork, or lamb—almost any meat, for that matter. A combination of hard sear (restaurant talk for deep browning) followed by slow cooking is the common denominator. The classic versions would have more meat and fewer vegetables, but with this technique and the slow oven braising, I think it's actually better this way.

12 ounces boneless chuck steak

2 tablespoons olive oil

1½ teaspoons salt

½ teaspoon pepper

1 onion, chopped

2 green bell peppers, chopped

4 celery stalks, chopped

1 pound button mushrooms, sliced

1 tablespoon minced garlic

1 tablespoon chopped fresh thyme, or 1 teaspoon dried

¼ teaspoon cayenne, more or less

One 28-ounce can whole peeled tomatoes

½ cup beef or vegetable stock (see page 246), or water, or more as needed

1 cup grits (not instant)

1 tablespoon butter

½ cup chopped fresh parsley, for garnish

1 Heat the oven to 250°F. Cut the steak against the grain into long slices, no more than ½ inch thick. Put the oil in a large ovenproof pot over medium-high heat. When it's hot, add some of the meat, working in batches to avoid crowding. Reserve ½ teaspoon salt and sprinkle each batch of the meat with a pinch of the remaining 1 teaspoon and some of the pepper. Cook until the meat is browned on all sides, adjusting the heat and turning the pieces as needed so they don't burn, 5 to 10 minutes for each batch. As they brown, transfer them to a platter. Repeat until all the meat is cooked.

2 Pour off all but 3 tablespoons of the fat if necessary and lower the heat to medium. Add the onion, bell peppers, celery, mushrooms, garlic, thyme, and cayenne. Cook, stirring occasionally, until the vegetables begin to soften, 5 to 10 minutes. Stir in the tomatoes and their juices and the stock, scraping up any browned bits from the bottom of the pot, then add the browned meat. The meat and vegetables should be about halfway submerged in braising liquid; if not, add more liquid until they are.

3 Raise the heat and bring to a boil, then lower it so that the mixture barely bubbles. Cover the pot and transfer it to the oven. Cook, stirring every 30 minutes, until the meat is fork-tender, at least 90 minutes and possibly as much as 2½ hours. As you stir, add another spoonful of liquid only if the pot looks too dry.

4 When the grillades are almost ready, put the grits in a medium pot with 1 cup water and whisk to form a smooth slurry. Whisk in ½ cup of the reserved stock and the remaining ½ teaspoon salt and set the pot over medium-high heat. Bring the mixture to a boil, then lower the heat so it bubbles gently but steadily; cook the grits, whisking frequently and adding more water a little at a time to prevent lumps and keeping the mixture somewhat soupy, 20 to 25 minutes. Expect to add another 2½ to 3½ cups of water before the grits are ready. They'll be thick and creamy, with just a little grittiness, and the mixture will pull away from the sides of the pan as you stir when they're done. Stir in the butter.

5 Taste and adjust the seasoning of both the grillades and the grits, then spoon the grits into shallow bowls, top with the stew, garnish with the parsley, and serve.

VARIATIONS

GRITS AND PORTABELLO GRILLADES Presto: vegan. Omit the meat and button mushrooms, and thinly slice 4 large portabello mushroom caps and stems. In Step 1, again working in batches, brown the portabello slices on both sides. (This will take much longer than the meat; figure as much as 20 minutes to do them all.) Follow the recipe, except in Step 3 reduce the cooking time to just long enough for the tomatoes to break down and the sauce to thicken, 10 to 15 minutes.

GRITS AND PORK GRILLADES Use thinly sliced pork shoulder instead of beef and sliced cabbage instead of the mushrooms.

MORE IDEAS

Add even more vegetables to the pot with the mushrooms: carrots, winter squash, cauliflower, or parsnips are all good choices. • Or add spinach, watercress, or other greens to the pot when you start the grits in Step 4. • Ratchet up the seasoning with chopped fresh red chiles; add them with the other vegetables in Step 2.

VEGETABLE CURRY WITH LAMB

MAKES 4 to 6 servings   **TIME** 1 to 2 hours, mostly unattended

A classic curry—with lots of vegetables—is far simpler to make than you might think. Just brown the meat; add the vegetables, stock, and aromatics; and let it simmer on the stove—it does its thing while you do yours. This reheats beautifully too, making it the ideal meal for weeknight entertaining or freezing for ready-to-eat suppers on hectic nights. Serve it with the bread on page 249 or brown rice (basmati is best here).

2 tablespoons vegetable oil

1 pound boneless lamb shoulder, cut into 1-inch chunks

1 teaspoon salt

½ teaspoon pepper

1 large onion, halved and sliced

1 red bell pepper, chopped

1 zucchini, chopped

1 small head cauliflower (about 1 pound), chopped

1 tablespoon minced garlic

1 tablespoon minced fresh ginger, or 1 teaspoon ground dried

2 tablespoons curry powder

½ teaspoon cayenne (optional)

2 cups chicken or vegetable stock (see page 246) or water, or more as needed

½ cup Greek yogurt

½ cup chopped fresh cilantro leaves, for garnish

1 Put the oil in a large pot over medium-high heat. When it's hot, add some of the lamb and sprinkle with some of the salt and pepper. Cook, adjusting the heat and turning the pieces as needed so the meat doesn't burn, until it's well browned on all sides, 5 to 10 minutes. As the meat browns, transfer it to a plate and continue adding more meat, seasoning it, and cooking the pieces until all the meat is browned.

2 Pour off all but 2 tablespoons of the fat and turn the heat down to medium. Add the onion, bell pepper, zucchini, cauliflower, garlic, and ginger, and cook, stirring occasionally, until the vegetables begin to soften, 5 to 10 minutes. Add the curry powder and cayenne, if you're using it, and cook, stirring constantly, until fragrant, 1 or 2 minutes.

3 Stir in the stock, scraping up any browned bits from the bottom of the pot, then add the browned lamb: The meat and vegetables should be about halfway submerged in braising liquid; if not, add more liquid. Bring to a boil, then lower the heat so the mixture barely bubbles. Cover and cook, stirring every 30 minutes and adding small amounts of liquid if the stew ever looks dry, until the meat is tender enough to cut with a fork, another 15 to 30 minutes.

4 If the curry looks too watery, remove the lid, raise the heat a bit, and cook, stirring frequently, until it thickens. If it looks too dry, add a little more stock or water and raise the heat until bubbly. Remove from the heat. Stir in the yogurt. Taste and adjust the seasoning, then garnish with the cilantro and serve.

VARIATION

CHILI BEEF WITH LOTS OF VEGETABLES Swap boneless beef chuck for the lamb, olive oil for the vegetable oil, and chili powder for the curry. Try carrots instead of the cauliflower and add 2 chopped poblano chiles along with the bell pepper. Omit the yogurt. Go ahead and add dried black beans with the stock in Step 3 if you like, but I bet you won't miss them. Serve with warm corn tortillas.

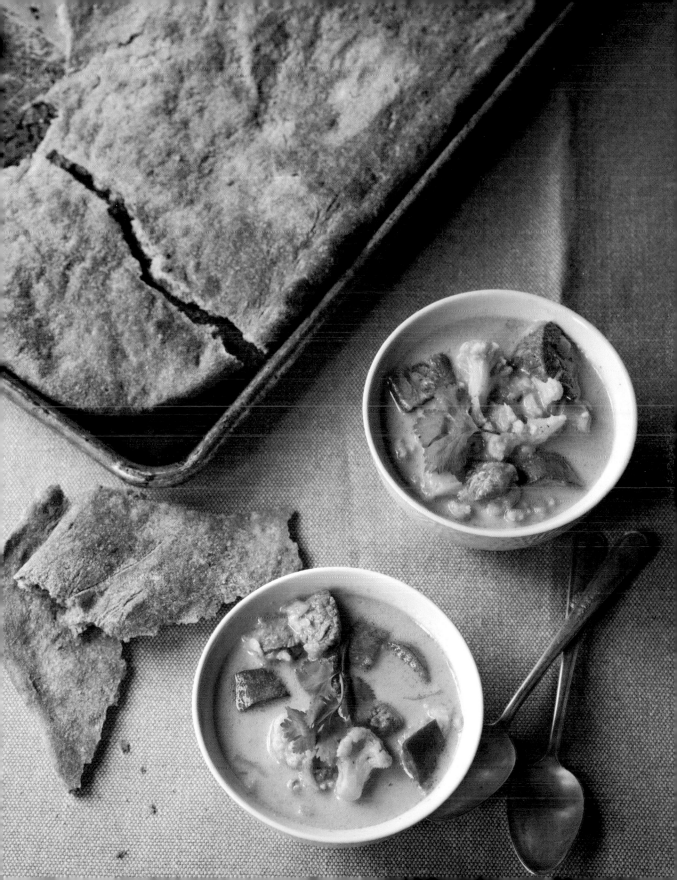

DESSERTS

TROPICAL FRUIT PUDDING

BALSAMIC FIGS

SUMMER PUDDING WITH
VANILLA CREAM

BANANA-CHOCOLATE ICE CREAM

PEANUT BUTTER BONBONS

AVOCADO CHOCOLATE MOUSSE

PEARS WITH CRISP TOPPING

DECADENT OATMEAL COOKIES

CHERRY CLAFOUTIS

RICE PUDDING WITH
SLOW-ROASTED FRUIT

No question: There's bliss in indulgence. Dessert, for many, is an essential pleasure at day's end. But you also want to be mindful of your hedonism: Savoring a few bites of something is almost always as good as—if not better than—gobbling a huge portion.

There's a middle ground on desserts, and I identify it here. These recipes aren't so packed with sugar or butter that you need to feel guilty about eating them—in fact, the vast majority are vegan, or nearly so—but they're decadent enough to feel like treats. Fruits, whole grains, and nuts are the primary stars, with chocolate, cream, and butter playing supporting roles. Or not. I have also thrown in a handful of pure VB6 wild cards, like avocados, nut butters, whole wheat flour, and silken tofu. When it comes to sweeteners I mainly use honey, maple syrup, and turbinado sugar—the latter being a raw, less processed sugar. Scan the ingredients list to see when non-vegan foods might come into play; wherever appropriate, I suggest possible substitutions after the recipe.

These are not fake diet-y desserts: They're fruity, creamy, or chocolaty enough to satisfy every kind of sweet tooth. And because you make them yourself—often literally in minutes—they're better for you than anything you'll find in the supermarket aisles. The recipes are also full of ideas for adapting the ingredients as the seasons change. You can incorporate different fruits or herbs, or try a new variation in the Banana-Chocolate Ice Cream (page 208) or the Cherry Clafoutis (page 217), depending on what's in your market. Of course, treats like Decadent Oatmeal Cookies (page 214) and Peanut Butter Bonbons (page 210) are always in season.

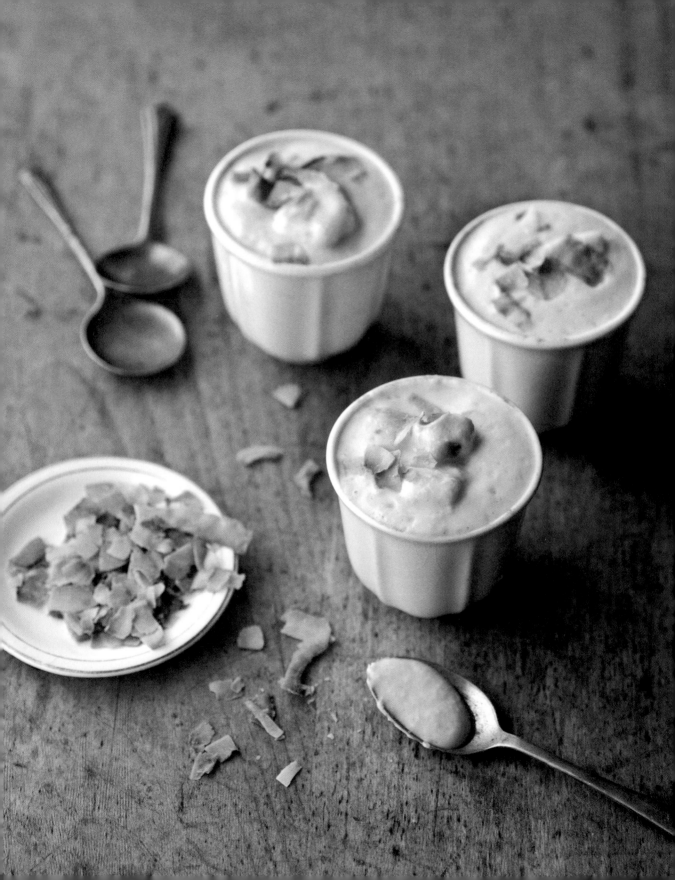

TROPICAL FRUIT PUDDING

MAKES 4 Servings   TIME 30 minutes, plus time to chill

Whenever I serve tofu pudding—and with so many variations I can make it frequently—everyone is shocked to find there's no dairy involved. Creamy and sweet with fresh mango, crunchy with toasted coconut, and bright with pineapple, this version is a great way to make tofu converts of your friends and family.

2 tablespoons maple syrup or other sweetener

24 ounces silken tofu (about 3 cups)

2 mangos, peeled, pitted, and cut into big chunks

½ teaspoon vanilla extract

⅛ teaspoon salt

¼ teaspoon coconut extract (optional)

½ large pineapple, peeled, quartered, and cored

¾ cup unsweetened shredded coconut

1   Put the syrup, tofu, mangos, vanilla, salt, and coconut extract, if you're using it, in a food processor or blender. Puree, stopping to scrape down the sides whenever necessary, until completely smooth, at least 1 minute total. Transfer the puree to a large bowl.

2   Chop the pineapple into ⅛ inch pieces and fold it into the pudding; cover the bowl tightly, and refrigerate for at least 30 minutes or up to several hours.

3   Put the coconut in a large skillet over medium heat. Cook, stirring frequently, until golden brown, 5 to 10 minutes. Remove from the oven and let cool. (You can store the coconut in an airtight container in the fridge for days.) To serve, spoon the pudding into bowls and sprinkle with the toasted coconut.

VARIATIONS

GINGERY MANGO PUDDING Ripe papaya—instead of the mango—is good this way too. Substitute ¼ cup minced candied ginger for the coconut. No need to toast; proceed directly to Step 2.

CHOCOLATE-CHERRY-COCONUT PUDDING Skip the mango, and use 2 cups chopped pitted cherries instead of the pineapple (frozen is fine; let thaw a bit first). Melt 6 ounces chopped dark chocolate and puree it with the tofu mixture in Step 2.

MORE IDEAS

Mix and match the fruits, changing both the pureed fruit and the chopped fruit. Some good combos are bananas with strawberries, peaches with raspberries, papaya with blueberries, and blueberries with peaches. You get the idea. • Top the pudding with toasted nuts instead of coconut.

BALSAMIC FIGS

MAKES 4 servings **TIME** 20 minutes, plus more time for macerating

Nothing beats the sweet suppleness of fresh figs. It really doesn't take much to turn them into a sophisticated dessert that is sure to be a crowd-pleaser—just a little marinating. And it's the easiest recipe in the chapter. Chances are you won't even need the sugar in the marinade, so try it without; you can always add it later.

¾ cup chopped walnuts

½ cup balsamic vinegar

¼ teaspoon salt

2 tablespoons sugar, preferably turbinado (optional)

1 pound fresh figs, green or black, halved

1 cup Greek yogurt

2 tablespoons honey

1 Put a small skillet over medium-low heat. Add the walnuts and cook, shaking the pan frequently until fragrant and lightly toasted, 3 to 5 minutes. Remove from the pan and let cool.

2 Combine the vinegar, salt, and sugar, if you're using it, in a large bowl and stir until the sugar is dissolved. Add the figs and toss gently with a rubber spatula until they're coated in marinade. Let sit at room temperature, stirring every once in a while, for at least 10 minutes or up to 30. (Or if you prefer to serve the fruit cold, let it sit in the fridge.)

3 Meanwhile, whisk the yogurt and honey together in a small bowl. When the figs are softened but not yet falling apart, spoon them into bowls with a slotted spoon. Top with the yogurt, a drizzle of the soaking liquid, and some chopped walnuts, and serve.

VARIATIONS

PORT-MARINATED FIGS For something even a bit more upscale, skip the sugar and use tawny or ruby port instead of the vinegar.

BALSAMIC STRAWBERRIES WITH BLACK PEPPER AND RICOTTA The classic from which all others come. Toast almonds, not walnuts. Instead of the sugar, use 1 tablespoon freshly ground black pepper. Swap fresh ricotta cheese for the yogurt, and mix the honey into it with a fork before serving.

BOOZY PINEAPPLE WITH MAPLE YOGURT Try pecans instead of walnuts. Use bourbon (or a mixture of bourbon and water or white balsamic vinegar) instead of the dark balsamic vinegar, and maple syrup instead of the sugar and honey. For even more kick, add a chopped fresh red chile (or a pinch of red chile flakes) to the marinade.

MORE IDEAS

Vary the nuts: In addition to those in the variations, pistachios, hazelnuts, cashews, and unsweetened shredded or sliced coconut are all good choices.
• Try ½ cup fresh goat cheese instead of the yogurt.

SUMMER PUDDING
WITH VANILLA CREAM

MAKES 4 servings   **TIME** 20 minutes, plus at least 8 hours to chill

A simple solution for dressing up juicy berries is to turn them into a summer pudding that's not only classic in flavor but also a healthy dessert option. Cutting the cream with silken tofu makes the perfect topping, but if you're feeling more decadent, just whip up a cup or so of cream.

1¾ pounds strawberries, raspberries, or blueberries, or a mix of all three, fresh or frozen

3 tablespoons honey

⅛ teaspoon nutmeg (optional)

6 or 7 slices bread, preferably whole grain

½ cup heavy cream

4 ounces silken tofu (about ½ cup)

1 teaspoon vanilla extract

1 If you're using strawberries, slice them; all other berries can remain whole. Combine the berries, honey, and nutmeg, if you're using it, with 1 tablespoon water in a saucepan over medium-high heat. Cook, stirring occasionally, until the fruit softens and releases its liquid, 3 to 5 minutes. Immediately drain, reserving the liquid, and let cool.

2 Meanwhile, cut the crusts off the bread. Line a 1-quart bowl with 5 or more of the slices; pack and cut them as necessary so they leave no (significant) gaps. Spoon the berries on top of the bread and drizzle with about two thirds of the liquid. Top the berries with enough of the remaining 1 or 2 slices of bread to cover them, again packing and cutting them for a close fit. Drizzle the remaining liquid on top.

3 Find a plate that fits into the bowl and press it down on top of the pudding. Weight it with a can (or whatever presses on the pudding a little) and put this rig inside a larger bowl to catch any overflowing juices. Refrigerate the whole thing for at least 8 hours or overnight.

4 When you're ready to serve, put the cream in a clean metal or glass bowl and beat with an electric mixer or a whisk until if forms firm peaks; be careful not to overbeat or it will separate into clumps. In another bowl, beat or whisk the tofu and vanilla. Fold the whipped cream into the tofu just until there are no streaks. Run a knife around the inside edge of the bowl and invert the pudding onto a plate. Cut slices and serve with the topping.

VARIATIONS

ANGEL FOOD CAKE SUMMER PUDDING For a more decadent alternative, substitute angel food cake slices for the bread slices.

GROWN-UP SUMMER PUDDING Substitute 2 tablespoons sherry, cream sherry, or port for some of the water in Step 1.

MORE IDEAS

Use any juicy fruit you have on hand, like mangos, peaches, plums, or figs. Cut them up into bite-size wedges, chunks, or slices.

BANANA-CHOCOLATE ICE CREAM

MAKES 4 servings   TIME 10 minutes, plus time to freeze

Besides making the smoothest smoothies, frozen bananas can be the basis for an amazing and *über*-versatile vegan ice cream (see photograph on page 215). The options are endless: Check out all of the variations below. If you have bananas in the freezer all the time, you can make this in a jiffy. Just peel and slice them; see page 51. Otherwise you'll need to plan a couple hours in advance.

4 ripe bananas, frozen and sliced

1 tablespoon unsweetened cocoa

2 tablespoons unsweetened plain non-dairy milk, or more as needed

½ teaspoon vanilla extract

⅛ teaspoon salt

3 ounces dark chocolate, chopped into chunks

1   Put the bananas in a food processor and puree until smooth, or nearly so; then add the cocoa, milk, vanilla, and salt. Pulse a few more times to combine. If the mixture seems too thick for the machine to handle add more milk a teaspoon at a time, but be careful not to thin the mixture too much; it should be spoonable, not pourable.

2   Remove the blade from the work bowl and fold in the chocolate with a rubber spatula. Transfer the mixture to an airtight container and freeze until solid (or nearly so), at least 2 hours. (It will keep for a couple of months but won't last that long.)

VARIATIONS

BANANA-MANGO ICE CREAM Replace one of the bananas with 1 chopped and frozen mango. Skip the cocoa powder and chocolate. In Step 1, blend the frozen banana and mango together. In Step 2, stir in ¼ cup shredded unsweetened coconut or chopped fresh mint (or both), if you'd like.

BANANA-CHOCOLATE-HAZELNUT ICE CREAM Before Step 1, chop ½ cup toasted hazelnuts in the food processor; remove and reserve them. Use hazelnut milk and skip the vanilla. In Step 2, stir in the nuts.

BANANA CREAM PIE ICE CREAM Omit the cocoa and chocolate. Before Step 1, chop 1 ounce graham crackers or vanilla wafers in the food processor (or about ¼ cup); remove and reserve them. Use cream instead of non-dairy milk if you'd like, and increase the vanilla to 1 tablespoon.

BANANA-PINEAPPLE-COCONUT ICE CREAM Freeze 1 cup chopped pineapple. Skip the cocoa powder and chocolate, and use coconut milk (reduced fat is fine). In Step 1, blend the frozen banana and pineapple together. In Step 2, stir in ¼ cup shredded unsweetened coconut.

BANANA-PISTACHIO-CARDAMOM ICE CREAM Skip the cocoa. Before
Step 1, chop ½ cup shelled pistachios in the food processor; remove and
reserve them. Add ¼ teaspoon ground cardamom with the vanilla in
Step 1. Stir in the nuts instead of the chocolate in Step 2.

MORE IDEAS

Leave out the cocoa and chocolate and just puree the frozen bananas and
other ingredients. • Add other fruits; melons, berries, and cherries are especially good. Buy them frozen or cut them up and freeze them yourself. • Go a
little decadent and use cream instead of the non-dairy milk. (See the Banana
Cream Pie variation on page 208.) • Add ½ teaspoon cinnamon in Step 1—and
keep the cocoa and chocolate or not.

BUYING CHOCOLATE

The snap of a high-quality bar when you break it and release the
aroma is intoxicating—even before you take a bite. The only thing
you really need to know about choosing good chocolate is this:
The higher the percentage of cocoa solids, the less sugar and milk
solids it will contain. High-cocoa chocolate is more expensive, but
it's worth it; even average supermarket brands now report their
percentage of cocoa on the label. Milk and white chocolates are
creamier, of course, but for flavor (and the reputed health benefits),
eat close to the bean.

PEANUT BUTTER BONBONS

MAKES 4 servings   TIME 15 minutes, plus time to freeze

These bite-size treats are different from the frozen truffle variation with banana on page 151 and more like a true peanut butter cup—quite cool. Don't be put off by the precision of the chocolate tempering here; it's not at all difficult.

1 cup peanut butter

¼ cup coconut milk (reduced-fat is fine), plus more as needed

¼ teaspoon salt

2 cups puffed brown rice cereal

8 ounces dark chocolate, chopped into small pieces

1 Line a rimmed baking sheet with parchment paper or foil. Combine the peanut butter, milk, and salt in a large bowl and whisk until smooth.

2 Add the rice cereal and stir until it's coated and softens, 1 or 2 minutes. Pinch it to see if it holds together easily; if not, add more milk, a little at a time. With two spoons or your hands, form the mixture into sixteen 1-inch balls. Refrigerate them while you make the chocolate (or covered in plastic for up to a day).

3 Melt 6 ounces of the chocolate in a small, clean metal or glass bowl set over gently bubbling water, or in the top of a double boiler. When the chocolate reaches between 110 and 115°F on a candy thermometer, remove the bowl from the heat.

4 Add the remaining chocolate to the bowl, stirring constantly with a rubber spatula until the chocolate reaches 82 to 84°F. Put the bowl back over the water and bring the temperature up to between 88 and 91°F.

5 Remove the chocolate from the heat and start dipping the bonbons: Use a fork to first coat each bonbon, then give it a twirl and turn it upside down so the peanut butter mixture is almost entirely covered. Put each piece on the prepared baking sheet to set the coating.

6 Repeat with the remaining chocolate and peanut butter balls, keeping the thermometer close by so you can keep checking the temperature. If it drops below 88°F (which it probably will once or twice), put the bowl back over the bubbling water until it returns to the 88 to 91°F range, then continue dipping. Refrigerate the bonbons until they're firm, then transfer them to an airtight container and refrigerate for up to a few days (or freeze for a couple of months).

MORE IDEAS

Use white chocolate instead of dark for dipping the peanut butter. • Use almond butter, cashew, or walnut butter instead of peanut butter. • Add ½ cup chopped dried cherries, cranberries, or raisins to the peanut butter mixture in Step 1. • Roll the bonbons in shredded, unsweetened coconut—toasted or not. • Use puffed millet instead of rice; it retains a little crunch.

AVOCADO CHOCOLATE MOUSSE

MAKES 4 servings   TIME 30 minutes, plus time to cool

Unlike a traditional mousse that uses eggs and heavy cream to create a silky texture, here I use avocado, a naturally creamy base. This is best with Hass or other nonwatery types combined with a very dark chocolate (meaning it has a high percentage of cocoa solids; see page 209), though there are other options (see below). I use powdered sugar because it really is the best sweetener for the job—and there isn't much of it.

4 ounces dark chocolate, chopped

2 ripe avocados, chopped

1 cup unsweetened plain non-dairy milk

2 tablespoons powdered sugar

½ teaspoon vanilla extract

¼ teaspoon salt

1 pint raspberries

1 Melt the chocolate in a small, clean metal or glass bowl set over gently bubbling water, or in the top of a double boiler. When it's almost completely melted, remove the bowl from the heat and stir the chocolate until it's completely smooth, about 1 minute. Let it cool until you can hold the bowl.

2 Transfer the chocolate to a large bowl with the remaining ingredients, and beat with an electric mixer until smooth and fluffy, 3 to 5 minutes. Refrigerate the mousse until cold—for at least 2 hours or up to several, but no more. Serve with the raspberries scattered on top.

VARIATIONS

MEXICAN CHOCOLATE AVOCADO MOUSSE A taste that I've definitely acquired. Use rice milk for the liquid and brown sugar instead of powdered sugar. Add ¼ teaspoon cayenne or other ground red chile and add ½ teaspoon ground cinnamon to the mixture in Step 2. Serve with chopped mangos instead of the raspberries.

CHOCOLATE COCONUT AVOCADO MOUSSE Stunningly similar to a Mounds bar in flavor. Start by toasting ½ cup unsweetened shredded coconut in a dry skillet. Use coconut milk (reduced-fat is fine) for the liquid and rum instead of vanilla, if you'd like. Garnish the mousse with the raspberries and toasted coconut.

CHOCOLATE ALMOND AVOCADO MOUSSE Start by toasting ½ cup chopped almonds in a dry skillet. Use almond milk for the liquid and almond liqueur instead of vanilla, if you'd like. Garnish the mousse with the raspberries and toasted almonds.

MORE IDEAS

Make this a bigger treat: Use regular milk, half-and-half, or cream instead of the non-dairy milk. • Garnish with chopped pecans, walnuts, or almonds. • Serve with strawberries or other berries.

PEARS WITH CRISP TOPPING

MAKES 4 servings   TIME 40 minutes

Good pears aren't in season for long, but when they are you should make this supremely easy and delicious dessert. (When they aren't, there are other fruits you can use; ideas are listed below. Normally I would suggest that frozen fruit is a fine substitute but here it's not.)

Pitting the pears is easy if they're "freestones": Cut the fruit downward from the stem, then scoop the seeds and core out with a melon baller, spoon, or paring knife. This technique works for apples too.

3 tablespoons butter, softened

1 tablespoon vegetable oil

¼ cup sugar, preferably turbinado

½ cup rolled oats (not quick-cooking or instant)

¼ cup whole wheat flour

¼ cup chopped walnuts

1 tablespoon fresh lemon juice

¼ teaspoon salt

4 large or 6 medium pears (about 2 pounds), halved, pitted, and seeds removed (see the headnote)

½ cup Greek yogurt (optional)

1 Use 2 teaspoons butter to grease a 9 by 13-inch baking dish. Cream the remaining butter, the oil, and the sugar with an electric mixer or fork. Add the oats, flour, walnuts, lemon juice, and salt and stir until combined. (You can make the topping ahead to this point, tightly wrap, and refrigerate for up to a day or freeze for up to several weeks; thaw before proceeding.)

2 Heat the oven to 400°F. Put the pear halves in the prepared dish and crumble the oats mixture on top. Bake until the pears are golden and the topping is just starting to brown, 25 to 35 minutes. If you're using the yogurt, beat it with a small spoon until smooth and a little fluffy. Serve right away, or at least while still warm, with the yogurt if you like.

VARIATIONS

FRUIT CRISP Good for berries and fruit that can't be halved easily. Figure about 1½ pounds: Plums, peaches, apples, nectarines, and figs will all work great. Use an 8- or 9-inch square pan instead and cut the fruit into 1-inch wedges or chunks (leave berries whole). Crumble the topping over all and bake as described in Step 2.

GRAPEFRUIT WITH SPICED CRISP TOPPING Better than broiled. Cut the grapefruit in half around the equator; cut the flesh free from the membrane with a paring or grapefruit knife, but leave the sections in the peel. Add ½ teaspoon each ground coriander and freshly ground black pepper to the topping.

APPLES WITH CRISP MAPLE TOPPING The classic for crisps. Substitute maple syrup for the sugar. Add 1 teaspoon of ground cinnamon to the topping.

PEACHES WITH PRALINE TOPPING A little sweeter, with a gooey candy-like crust. Omit the flour and instead of the walnuts use pecans; increase the sugar to ⅓ cup. Substitute peaches for the pears; halve them around the equator and remove the pits. Top and bake the fruit as directed.

PINEAPPLE WITH COCONUT-CASHEW TOPPING You've got to use fresh fruit here; it takes only a few minutes to prepare. Use unsweetened shredded coconut instead of the oats, and cashews instead of walnuts, and add ½ teaspoon cardamom to the topping, if you'd like. Trim and peel 1 large pineapple. Cut it lengthwise into quarters and remove the core from each piece; then slice the quarters thinly enough so they almost lay flat. In Step 1, spread the pineapple into the prepared dish, then top and bake as directed.

MORE IDEAS

Stir 2 tablespoons of minced ginger into the crumble topping before baking • Use lime or orange juice instead of the lemon juice. • Rice flour makes this very delicate: Substitute brown rice flour for the wheat flour. • Swap any other nut (or unsweetened shredded coconut) for the walnuts. • Go vegan: Use 3 tablespoons oil instead of the butter (for a total of ¼ cup vegetable oil). Instead of the yogurt topping, whisk 1 cup silken tofu until it's smooth and spoon that over the warm crisp.

DECADENT OATMEAL COOKIES

MAKES 1 dozen cookies   TIME About 30 minutes, plus time to cool

This recipe makes a dozen good-sized, fully loaded—*packed*—
whole-grain, fun-to-eat treats. Yes, there's sugar and fat in them; that's
what makes them worth eating. And the darker the chocolate—meaning
the higher percentage of cocoa solids (see page 209)—the better. Serve
these with Banana-Chocolate Ice Cream (page 208) for true decadence.

¼ cup vegetable oil

½ cup sugar, preferably turbinado

2 tablespoons unsweetened applesauce

¾ cup whole wheat flour

1 cup rolled oats (not quick-cooking or instant)

¼ teaspoon salt

1 teaspoon baking powder

¼ cup unsweetened plain non-dairy milk

½ teaspoon vanilla extract

¼ cup chopped walnuts or pecans

½ cup dried cherries or cranberries, chopped

2 tablespoons unsweetened shredded coconut

2 ounces dark chocolate, chopped into small chunks

1   Heat the oven to 375°F. Beat together the oil, sugar, and applesauce in a small bowl with an electric mixer until fluffy, about 2 minutes.

2   Combine the flour, oats, salt, and baking powder in a large bowl. Add the sugar mixture, the milk, and vanilla, and mix on low until just blended. Fold in the nuts, fruit, coconut, and chocolate chunks with a rubber spatula.

3   Form 12 cookies with a spoon and drop them about 3 inches apart onto an ungreased baking sheet; press down lightly to flatten. Bake until lightly browned on the bottom, 12 to 15 minutes. Cool for about 2 minutes on the sheets, then carefully transfer the cookies to a wire rack with a spatula to cool completely. (Store in a tightly covered container at room temperature for no more than 1 or 2 days; after that freeze them.)

VARIATIONS

NOT VEGAN OATMEAL COOKIES The traditional way, so they're even more decadent. Make any or all of the following substitutions: use 4 tablespoons (½ stick) softened unsalted butter instead of oil; 1 egg instead of the applesauce; cow's milk instead of the non-dairy milk.

VEGAN (OR NOT) CHOCOLATE CHUNK OATMEAL COOKIES Keep it simple. Double the chocolate and leave out the nuts, dried fruit, and shredded coconut.

MORE IDEAS

You can use brown sugar instead of turbinado for a little different kind of sweet flavor. • Try adding up to 2 teaspoons ground instant espresso or coffee to the dry ingredients in Step 2. • Substitute dark raisins, golden raisins, or currants for the dried fruit. • Vary the nuts; pecans, hazelnuts, and pistachios are all good. • Instead of some or all of the oats, use crumbled shredded wheat cereal for a terrific change of flavor and texture. • Make bars: Press the mixture into a greased 8- or 9-inch square pan and bake as directed. Let the pan cool entirely before cutting them into 12 or 16 bars. Or bake bars for a crowd: Double the batch and press into a 9 by 13-inch pan.

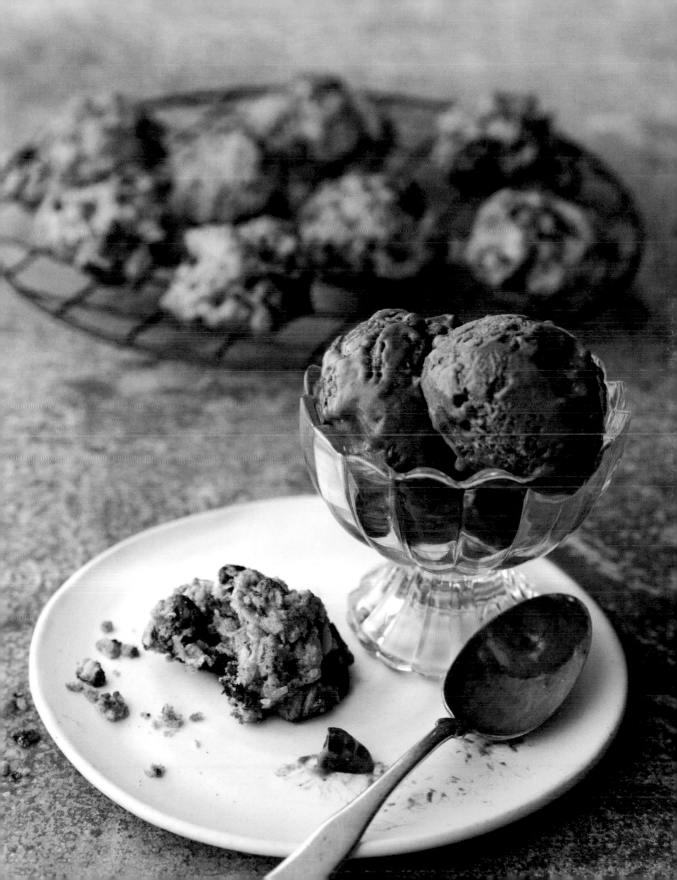

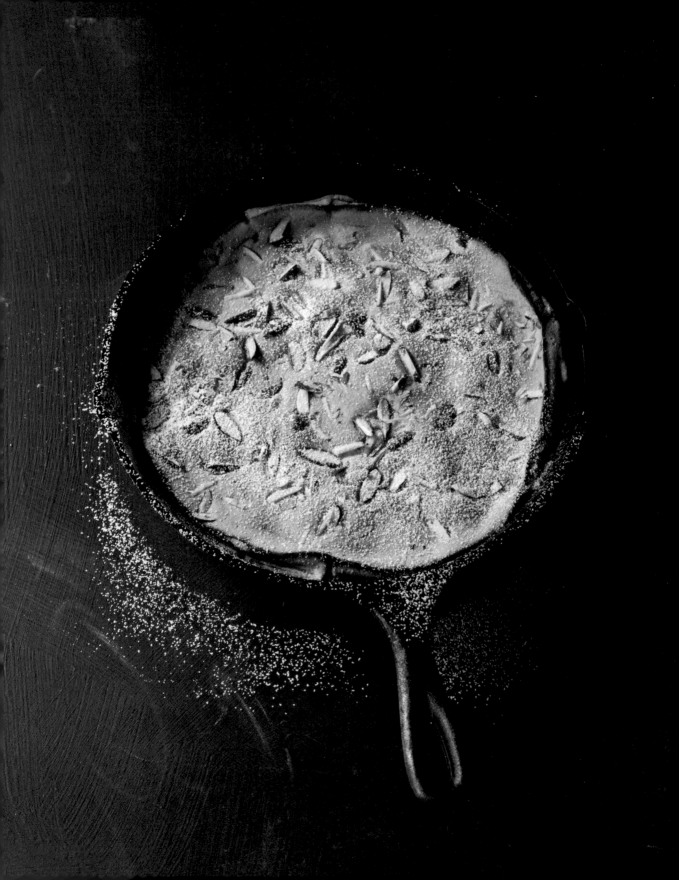

CHERRY CLAFOUTIS

MAKES 4 servings   TIME About 40 minutes

The French *clafoutis* (pronounced cla-FOO-tee) is a bit like a dessert
frittata, a cross between a flan and a fruit pancake. I give the traditional
recipe a makeover here by using more fruit and less batter. Beating the
egg whites helps you get the most from just a few eggs and makes them
bake more like a soufflé topping. And though cherries are the traditional
clafoutis fruit, you have lots of options; see the variations that follow.

2 tablespoons butter

1 pound cherries, pitted,
halved if you like

2 eggs, separated

¼ cup all-purpose white
flour

¾ cup any milk

1 teaspoon vanilla extract

¼ teaspoon salt

¼ cup sugar, preferably
turbinado

2 tablespoons chopped
almonds (optional)

2 tablespoons powdered
sugar, for dusting (optional)

1 Heat the oven to 375°F. Melt the butter in a large ovenproof skillet
over medium heat. When it foams, spread the cherries in the pan and
turn off the heat.

2 Put the egg whites in a small bowl. Put the yolks in a medium bowl
with the flour, milk, vanilla, and salt and whisk until smooth.

3 Beat the egg whites with an electric mixer until foamy. Add the
sugar and keep beating until stiff peaks form. Fold the whites into the
yolk mixture, working up gently from the bottom of the bowl with a
rubber spatula until the color is almost uniform; it's okay if there are
still some streaks.

4 Spoon the batter over the fruit, top with the almonds, if using, and
bake until the clafoutis is lightly browned and puffy on top and a knife
inserted into the center comes out clean, 20 to 30 minutes, depending on
the size of your skillet. Let it cool a bit. Sift confectioners' sugar over it
if you'd like, and serve warm or at room temperature.

VARIATIONS

GINGERED APRICOT CLAFOUTIS Omit the almonds. Substitute sliced
apricots for cherries and add 1 tablespoon grated ginger to the egg yolk
mixture in Step 2.

CINNAMON APPLE CLAFOUTIS Omit the almonds. Substitute chopped
apples for the cherries. In Step 1 when the butter foams, add 1 teaspoon
cinnamon to the skillet before adding the apples. Cook the apples in
the butter until they soften, 3 to 5 minutes. Then turn off the heat and
continue with the recipe.

BLUEBERRY-LEMON CLAFOUTIS Use blueberries, not cherries. Add
2 teaspoons grated lemon zest to the egg yolk mixture in Step 2.

MORE IDEAS

Almost any fruit can be used for clafoutis; in addition to the ones in the variations, try pears, peaches, nectarines, grapes, or plums.

RICE PUDDING WITH SLOW-ROASTED FRUIT

MAKES 4 servings   TIME About 2½ hours, largely unattended

This is a time-intensive dish, but it doesn't take much work at all, and it's worth every minute. For a thicker pudding, veer toward the high end of the rice quantities listed below. The trick is to crack the hard exterior of the rice—use a food processor for that—so that it releases its starch and thickens the pudding. And there's one more trick: patience. It won't look like pudding until it's out of the oven and rests.

⅓ to ½ cup long-grain brown rice (see the headnote)

3½ cups unsweetened plain non-dairy milk

⅓ cup sugar, preferably turbinado

½ teaspoon salt

4 peaches, peeled if you like, sliced

2 tablespoons olive oil

½ teaspoon ground cinnamon

1 Heat the oven to 300°F. Put the quantity of rice you want in a food processor and pulse a few times to break the grains up a bit and scratch their hulls. Don't overdo it, or you'll pulverize them; just pulse until you see some slight damage being done.

2 Put the rice in a 2-quart baking dish with the milk, sugar, and salt. Stir a couple of times and put the dish in the oven, uncovered. Cook for 45 minutes undisturbed, then stir. Let it cook undisturbed for another 45 minutes; then stir again. At this point the milk will have darkened a little and the rice will have begun to swell.

3 Meanwhile, spread the peaches on a rimmed baking sheet; drizzle with the oil, toss, then spread out again. Cook until they brown around the edges and release easily from the pan, 20 to 25 minutes. Sprinkle with the cinnamon, toss with a spatula, spread out again, and roast until caramelized, another 20 to 25 minutes. They're going to be ready before the pudding and that's fine; just let them sit and cool while it finishes.

4 After the pudding has cooked the initial 90 minutes, start stirring and checking it every 15 minutes, stirring gently each time. You're waiting for the milk to get even darker and for the pudding to start looking more like rice than milk. It might take as long as another 60 minutes for the pudding to be ready. Just trust your instincts and remove the pudding from the oven when it is still somewhat soupy; it will thicken a lot as it cools. Serve the pudding topped with the peaches, either warm or at room temperature.

CHOCOLATE-CHERRY BROWN RICE PUDDING Instead of roasting peaches, stir 2 cups pitted cherries into the pudding when you think you only have 30 minutes or so left to cook in Step 4. After the pudding has cooled a little but is still slightly warm, stir in 2 ounces chopped dark chocolate.

COCONUT-BROWN RICE PUDDING WITH PINEAPPLE Rich but still vegan. Use coconut milk (reduced-fat is fine). Toast ½ cup unsweetened shredded coconut in a dry skillet. When the pudding comes out of the oven, stir in the coconut.

RICHER BROWN RICE PUDDING WITH ROASTED PEACHES Veering toward decadent. Use low- or full-fat cow's milk instead of non-dairy and substitute melted butter for the olive oil.

THICK AND COLD RICE PUDDING The starch in the rice really seizes up when the pudding chills; for the thickest pudding, put it in the fridge for a couple hours or up to a couple days before serving.

MORE IDEAS

Roast other fresh fruits, like plums, mangos, pineapple, papayas, melons, or figs, instead of peaches. • Explore other spices: To season the peaches as they roast, try a pinch of saffron, ground cardamom, or ginger. • In Step 2, add 2 teaspoons grated lemon or orange zest. • About halfway through cooking, add ¼ cup raisins, dried berries, chopped dates, or chopped dried figs. • Just before serving, garnish the pudding with chopped nuts or chopped fresh mint or basil.

VB6
BUILDING
BLOCKS

Elemental as they are, these recipes are in many ways the book's most important element—the make-ahead basics that provide the foundation for a VB6 lifestyle (and, in a very real way, for basic cooking). If you start by preparing one of these every few days, you'll be taking a giant leap toward the real food and daily cooking that's at the heart of VB6.

You'll also be optimizing the time you spend in the kitchen, because it's almost always as easy to make a big batch of something as a small one, and to have it cooking unattended on a back burner while you prepare something else. Cooking components in bulk ensures that you're never scrambling to get dinner on the table or to pack a lunch to bring to work. With just a little advance planning you can eliminate the excuses for not making a change for the better in how you cook and eat.

In the process, you'll learn how to prepare, vary, and repurpose a handful of master recipes so that plant-based eating is neither boring nor difficult. Armed with staples like homemade sauces and seasonings, pots of grains and beans, simple fruit preparations, and a single recipe for how to cook almost every vegetable that exists, you'll find putting together your weekly meals a stress-free and pleasurable endeavor.

Consider this chapter an investment in your future. When you have salad ready to go, for example (see pages 224–226), you're more likely to eat salad; with a quart of stock in the freezer (see page 246), homemade soup is ready in a flash. And you'll learn the techniques and flavor combinations that will inspire your own ideas for creating a lifetime of VB6 meals and snacks.

FRUIT COMPOTE

MAKES 4 servings   **TIME** About 45 minutes

I eat a fair amount of fruit out of hand, but there are times when "doing something" to fruit makes it feel more like a treat. So here are three easy preparations that elevate fruit from snack to dish: compote, puree, and macerated (which essentially means marinated). The first two are cooked; the third just sits. Compotes and purees are the best ways to use fruit that's veering toward overripe; marinate fruit that's in its prime but not especially flavorful. If you skip the optional sugar, you can enjoy compote as an Unlimited Food; otherwise, put it in the Treats group. It's good on toast or with muffins or quick breads, stirred into grains, served as a sauce with plain cooked meats, or eaten with a spoon for a snack or dessert.

2 pounds fresh fruit, any kind (see More Ideas), one type or a mixture

½ teaspoon salt

¼ cup sugar, preferably turbinado (optional)

1　Trim, peel, pit, and/or seed the fruit as necessary. Cut it into 1- or 2- inch chunks or slices. Put ½ cup water in a large pot or skillet over medium heat; add the salt and the sugar, if you're using it. When the water begins to bubble, start adding the fruit, beginning with the firmest and adding the softer ones as the first begin to turn tender, so that the whole thing doesn't turn into mush. Adjust the heat so the mixture bubbles gently but steadily.

2　Cook, stirring occasionally and adding a splash if water if the mixture gets too dry, until the fruit is tender and the color darkens, 15 to 30 minutes, depending on the fruit. Serve warm or cool (or let the mixture chill completely and store in a jar in the refrigerator for up to a week).

VARIATIONS

PUREED FRUIT Once the fruit is tender, let it cool for a few minutes, then transfer it to a blender or food processor; puree until it reaches the texture you like.

MARINATED FRUIT No cooking necessary. Instead, combine the fruit, the sugar if you're using it, and the salt in a large bowl and stir until the sugar is dissolved. Add a squeeze of lemon, lime, or orange if you'd like. Toss gently with a rubber spatula until the fruit is coated in the marinade. Let sit at room temperature, stirring every once in a while, for at least 10 minutes or up to 30 minutes. (Or if you prefer to eat the fruit cold, let it sit in the fridge.)

SAVORY FRUIT, THREE WAYS Prepared fruit doesn't necessarily have to be sweet (think of salsa, page 236; or chutney). Once the fruit is prepared, you can add minced garlic, ginger, and chiles; dried spices like curry powder and ground cloves; or even a tiny splash of wine, soy sauce, vinegar, or hot sauce. Serve hot or cold, the same way you would fresh or cooked salsa.

MORE IDEAS

Almost any fruit will work, alone or in combination: apples, pears, peaches, nectarines, plums, cherries, berries, mangos, pineapple, even citrus. • For added flavor, squeeze in a pinch of citrus juice or sprinkle in some chopped fresh basil, mint, or even rosemary toward the end.

EVERYDAY SALAD BOWL

MAKES about four 3-cup servings   TIME 30 minutes

There's a reason why pre-washed greens and salad kits are so popular:
They're convenient. Making your own washed-and-ready greens at home
is only slightly less convenient, and they'll be infinitely fresher and totally
customizable. Properly stored, the components last for days in the fridge.

The goal is to have about 12 total cups prepared ingredients, enough
for four hearty salads. (If your household is full of salad eaters, double the
recipe.) Rinse, trim, and chop vegetables that don't discolor or wilt, like
celery, carrots, peppers, onions, cucumbers, or radishes, and keep them
in a bowl of water. Tear, rinse, dry, and store lettuce in a salad spinner
or in a plastic bag or airtight container lined with a towel. Keep a jar of
your own dressing (see page 226) handy in the fridge. A fresh side salad is
never more than a minute away; with a few additions, you've got a satisfying meal in a flash.

4 celery stalks

4 carrots

½ red onion

1 cucumber

1 red or green bell pepper

1 bunch radishes

1 large head romaine
lettuce

1 pint cherry or grape
tomatoes

Your Own Salad Dressing
(page 226)

1 Trim, peel, seed, or core the vegetables as necessary, as far in
advance as you want. Slice or chop them as you like; tear the lettuce
into bite-sized pieces. Store them as described in the headnote.

2 Combine as many ingredients as you like, and drizzle about
3 tablespoons of dressing per serving (about 3 cups) over all. Toss
and serve immediately.

VARIATIONS

EVERYDAY COOKED VEGETABLE SALAD Substitute any combination of
leftover cooked vegetables for the raw chopped vegetables and lettuce.
(Figure 2 cups per serving.) Drizzle with the dressing or a squeeze of
lemon; serve cold or at room temperature.

MORE IDEAS

Go with the season: Substitute root vegetables (turnips, rutabagas, or
beets) for the cucumbers; celery root for the celery; daikon or jícama for the
radishes; and apples, pears, or citrus for the tomato. Instead of lettuce, try
ribbons of cabbage (any kind) or raw kale or collards.

DON'T FORGET ABOUT FRUIT SALAD

I guarantee that if you have fruit cut up and ready to eat in the fridge, you will reach for it before you go for junk. What you want is a combination of fruits that hold up well for a couple of days; then you can add bananas, apples, peaches, nectarines, or pears (which all brown relatively quickly) as you serve it if you'd like.

The best-keeping cut fruits are mangos, papaya, pineapple, citrus, melons, plums, figs, grapes, kiwi, and berries. Figure about 3 pounds of any or all of these; trim and peel them as necessary, then cut them into no smaller than 1-inch pieces so they'll be less likely to disintegrate.

And don't be shy about seasoning fruit salad. A squeeze of citrus juice—I'm partial to lime—is always welcome, as is a pinch of salt. For something more exotic try a few grinds of black pepper or a sprinkling of cayenne or other ground chiles; even curry powder can work, especially with tropical fruits. Fresh herbs like mint, basil, rosemary, or lavender can add lovely floral notes; they'll discolor shortly after chopping so add them just before serving.

YOUR OWN SALAD DRESSING

MAKES 8 servings   **TIME** 10 minutes

I can't remember the last time I bought bottled dressing, but it was over 35 years ago. The stuff in stores is expensive at best (especially since the first ingredient is sometimes water) and loaded with sugar and chemicals at worst. Yet few things in life come together more quickly or more satisfyingly than homemade vinaigrette. Forget about fretting over whether the ingredients are emulsified (blended into a stable, uniform mixture). You just need it to stay blended long enough to pour. So put everything in a jar, shake it up, and use what you need, then close the lid, put it in the fridge, and shake again next time you're ready for a salad. It'll keep a week or so. For more about choosing the oil and vinegar, see the pantry listings on pages 23 and 31.

½ cup olive oil

½ cup any vinegar

¼ cup Dijon mustard

1 teaspoon dried thyme or tarragon (optional)

½ teaspoon salt, plus more to taste

Black pepper to taste

Put the oil, vinegar, mustard, and herb, if you're using it, in a 1-pint jar with a tight-fitting lid; add ¼ cup water, the salt, and some pepper. Shake vigorously until well combined. (Refrigerate for up to 1 week.)

VARIATIONS

YOUR OWN SOY DRESSING A perfect dipping or drizzling sauce for simply cooked meats, tofu, noodles, rice, or vegetables, as well as for salads. Use vegetable instead of olive oil. (In this recipe I like 6 or 7 tablespoons grapeseed or sunflower oil mixed with 1 or 2 tablespoons sesame oil.) Use rice vinegar if you have it. Skip the salt and start by adding 1 tablespoon soy sauce, then taste and adjust; keep the mustard if you'd like. For the herb, use ¼ cup fresh chopped cilantro, or add sesame seeds or ¼ teaspoon five-spice powder.

YOUR OWN CREAMY DRESSING Simply replace half the oil with something creamy, like yogurt, cream, or mayonnaise. For a vegan dressing, use silken tofu or Vegannaise (page 242).

YOUR OWN CAESAR DRESSING Not vegan, of course (unless you use Vegannaise, page 242), but necessary. Use this right away since it doesn't keep well (for that reason, this variation makes half as much as the main recipe). Put ¼ cup olive oil, ¼ cup lemon juice, and 2 tablespoons water in the jar. Add ¼ cup grated Parmesan cheese, 2 mashed anchovies, dash Worcestershire sauce, and one 2-minute soft-boiled egg. (If you're worried about the safety of undercooked eggs, use ¼ cup silken tofu or 2 tablespoons mayonnaise instead.) Skip the salt but add lots of black pepper. Shake, taste, and adjust the seasoning, then shake again. Chill for up to a couple hours if you'd like before serving.

BIG-BATCH COOKED VEGETABLES

MAKES 4 to 8 servings   TIME 10 to 30 minutes, depending on vegetable

You can cook pretty much any vegetable in bulk successfully and easily. The result can become tonight's side dish, play a role in dinner for a crowd, or help round out lunches during the week. This recipe covers it all, with guidelines for techniques that you can modify to work with what you like and have on hand. The main recipe is for versatile boiled vegetables, adaptable for how you plan to use them: crisp-tender or still a bit on the crunchy side for salads or stir-fries; fully tender, perfect for bowls of rice, noodles, or soups; or even "well done," for purees, sauces, soups, and spreads. If you're planning on cooking them ahead (for some undetermined meal in the future), go for undercooked vegetables. (You can't undo well-doneness.) It makes sense to boil only one kind of vegetable at a time, since different vegetables take longer to cook than others.

"Shocking" crisp-tender vegetables in an ice bath captures their color and doneness so you can use them in salads, stir-fries, or nibbling. Here's how: Fill a clean sink or large bowl with ice water. As soon as the vegetables soften just a little and their color becomes vibrant, quickly drain them and plunge them into the ice water; drain again, and wrap tightly to refrigerate or freeze for another time.

One last tip: If you want to eat the thick stems (sometimes called "ribs") of greens like chard, bok choy, kale, collards, and broccoli, separate them from the leaves (or florets, in the case of broccoli), peel if needed (again, in the case of broccoli), chop them roughly, and begin cooking them 2 or 3 minutes before you start the leaves (or florets)—this way everything will become tender at about the same time.

Cooked vegetables store well: You can refrigerate them in a covered container for a few days or freeze them for up to 1 month. Reheat them in a microwave, or warm them in some oil in a skillet for a couple of minutes.

Or eat them right away: Serve the vegetable drizzled with the lemon juice and oil, sprinkled with the remaining ½ teaspoon salt (or more) and some pepper; add the herbs or seasonings you like.

(recipe continues)

2 teaspoons salt, plus more
to taste

About 3 pounds vegetables,
virtually any kind except
peppers and eggplant

2 tablespoons fresh lemon
juice, plus more to taste

2 tablespoons olive oil

Black pepper to taste

Chopped fresh herbs
or ground seasonings
(optional)

1 Bring a large pot of water to a boil and add 1½ teaspoons salt. Trim, peel, stem, and seed the vegetables as needed, then cut into big chunks or slices if necessary. When the water boils, put the vegetables in the pot and cook uncovered.

2 Check tender greens after less than 1 minute; root vegetables will take 10 minutes or more. Everything else is somewhere in between. Every so often while the vegetables are cooking, pluck a piece out with tongs and test it. (With experience, you won't need to do this so often.) Remember that the vegetables will continue to cook a little as they cool.

3 When the vegetables are just a little bit more firm than you ultimately want them, transfer them to a colander to drain with a slotted spoon or tongs; then return the water in the pot to a boil before adding more vegetables. (This is the stage at which you'll shock them if you plan to do so; see headnote.)

VARIATIONS

STEAMED VEGETABLES For rigging a steamer, you're rewarded with less waterlogged vegetables: If you've got one of those collapsible steaming inserts (or a basket that fits into a covered pot like a double boiler), set it up, then add water to just below its base. To rig your own steamer, put about 1 inch of water in a large pot, then put a heatproof plate or bowl upside down in the bottom. Put another heatproof plate (pie plates are great for this if your pot is big enough) upright, on top. Add the food to the pot, cover, and turn the heat to high. Adjust the heat so the water bubbles steadily but not violently. If you're going to be cooking for more than a few minutes, be sure to peek inside and add water or adjust the heat as necessary.

MICROWAVE-COOKED VEGETABLES You'll need to cook this amount of vegetables in two batches. Put the vegetables on a plate or in a shallow bowl along with a few drops of water; don't drown them. Cover loosely with a paper towel, a vented microwave cooking lid, or a heavy plate. Set the timer for 5 minutes on high, but don't walk away: Timing will depend on your oven's power. Every 1 or 2 minutes, stop the machine and—careful of the steam—poke the vegetables with a thin-bladed knife to check for doneness. When the vegetables are cooked as you like them, proceed as above.

STIR-FRIED (SAUTÉED) VEGETABLES You can include peppers and eggplant in this method. For the best results, work in two or three batches. Put 2 tablespoons olive or vegetable oil in a large skillet over high heat. When it's hot, add the vegetables, about 1 pound at a time, and sprinkle with a little salt and pepper. Cook, stirring frequently, until they're just a little less tender than you ultimately want them (they'll continue to cook out of the pan). Add water, 2 tablespoons at a time, to help the vegetables soften evenly and keep them from sticking. Remove from the pan and repeat with the remaining vegetables.

ROASTED VEGETABLES Peppers and eggplant work here too. Heat the oven to 425°F. Spread the cut vegetables on one or two rimmed baking sheets. Drizzle them with 2 tablespoons olive or vegetable oil and sprinkle with salt and pepper; toss until coated. Cook, undisturbed, until they brown around the edges and release easily from the pan, 15 to 30 minutes, depending on the vegetable. Then toss with a spatula, scraping up any browned bits from the bottom of the pans. Continue to cook, tossing every once in a while, until the vegetables are as browned and tender as you want them, anywhere from 15 to 30 minutes more.

DRY-ROASTED VEGETABLES Takes little or no attention. This will also work well with peppers and eggplant. Trim the vegetables, but leave them whole if they're small; halve them if they're large and round. Heat the oven to 325°F. Put the cut vegetables on one or two rimmed baking sheets, cut side down if they're halved. Roast undisturbed until they're tender and browned on the bottom (they'll release fairly easily from the pan), anywhere from 45 to 90 minutes depending on the vegetable. Sprinkle with salt and pepper (and drizzle with olive or other oil) when you cut them up to serve or store.

PUT A LID ON IT

Cooking in big batches is a key strategy for simplifying VB6 cooking. If you will be cooking food ahead and storing it for future use, however, you might consider changing your approach to food storage. I try to avoid plastic containers whenever possible, as there are legitimate concerns about the safety of most plastics, especially during reheating. Glass and ceramic dishes and jars are more environmentally friendly and if you reuse jars, you already own some airtight containers.

For reheating, always make sure the vessel is intended for use in the microwave or oven. And whether you freeze in glass or plastic, be sure to leave "headroom": at least 1 inch of air at the top of the container to accommodate expansion as the food freezes. For more specific information on how long ingredients keep, see the charts that begin on pages 18, 26, and 35.

BIG-BATCH BROWN RICE AND WHOLE GRAINS

MAKES about 8 servings   **TIME** 10 minutes to more than 1 hour, depending on the grain

I can barely imagine a day without whole grains—that is, real whole grains, simply cooked in a pot of boiling water. The great thing is that I don't have to cook them every day to eat them every day—and neither will you. Like beans, they keep and reheat perfectly. So with this one recipe—which is really a formula, since it's so flexible—you can have homemade grains handy at all times.

It's almost impossible to mess up the method: If the pot cooks dry, you add a little more water. Started with too much water to the pot? Drain the grain like pasta. There's virtually no learning curve; one or two tries and you will know exactly what to look for.

And this technique works for virtually every grain: all kinds of brown and red rices, bulgur, quinoa, barley, steel-cut oats, farro, millet, cracked wheat, dried hominy or posole, wheat berries, and wild rice. (See the variation for how to cook couscous.) The larger the kernel, the longer it will take to become tender, but it's easy to monitor: Benchmarks and cues in the recipe will help you master the different cooking times and recognize doneness.

Once you have a batch ready, you can keep it for up to a week in the fridge. Use the grains in salads or soups, or reheat them in single or multiple servings as side dishes. Warm them in the microwave on medium, or in a covered pot on the stovetop with a few drops of water over low heat, or toss in a bit of oil to reheat. You can freeze them, too, for up to a few months: When you're ready, just thaw them in the fridge or microwave.

3 cups rice or whole grain (see the headnote for examples)

2 teaspoons salt, plus more to taste

1   Rinse the rice or grains in a strainer, then put them in a large pot with the salt. Add enough water to cover by about 1 inch, no more. Bring to a boil, then adjust the heat so the mixture bubbles gently.

2   Cover and cook undisturbed until the grains are tender and almost all of the water has been absorbed. This will take as little as 5 to 10 minutes for bulgur, 15 to 20 minutes for steel-cut oats, 20 to 25 minutes for quinoa and farro, at least 30 minutes for long-grain brown rice, and as long as 1 hour or more for some specialty rices and other sturdy grains like wheat berries or dried hominy. If the grains dry out before they're tender, add boiling water as needed to prevent them from sticking and scorching or burning.

3 Every now and then, taste a few grains; they're done when tender but still a little chewy. If the water is all absorbed (watch for the little holes that form on the surface), just cover the pot and remove it from the heat. If some water still remains but the grains are done, drain them in a strainer, return to the pot, cover, and remove from the heat. Undisturbed, they'll stay warm for about 20 minutes. To serve, fluff the grains with a fork. Serve as is or add flavorings.

VARIATIONS

BIG-BATCH WHOLE WHEAT COUSCOUS Actually, couscous is a very small pasta, but it cooks and eats more like a grain. As soon as the water comes to a boil in Step 1, cover the pot and remove it from the heat. Let it steep for at least 10 minutes or up to 20 minutes. Fluff with a fork and serve or store as you would any whole grain.

BIG-BATCH SOFT COOKED GRAINS Almost like mashed potatoes, grains cooked this way develop a pleasantly starchy texture; they're perfect for holding together burgers, meatballs, and savory cakes too. In Step 1, cover the grains with about 1½ inches of water and increase the cooking time by 5 minutes before you start checking and adding more water if they look too dry. Go ahead and stir them to make sure they're not sticking; you want to encourage them to stick together. They're ready when the water is absorbed and the kernels burst so the grains begin to form a single mass. Serve or store them the same as you would any whole grain.

MORE IDEAS

Whatever you can add to beans either before, during, or after cooking you can add to grains. For flavorings and seasonings, see the sidebar on page 234.

BIG-BATCH COOKED BEANS

MAKES about 8 servings   TIME 30 minutes to 2 hours, depending on bean and soaking option; largely unattended

The bean recipes in this cookbook always call for cooked or canned beans. The difference is simple: Canned beans are instant, but they also may taste tinny (or too salty); you can't control their texture (they're always soft, not necessarily a bad thing, but that's how it is); and they're relatively expensive. Dried beans take time to cook; other than that, they're just better in every way.

Try cooking dried beans yourself, and you might become a convert. Bear in mind that you can cook a big batch (as I do here) and have plenty of cooked beans at the ready for the rest of the week. And there's a bonus: You'll gain the cooking water, a liquid as flavorful as any broth with all the same value for soups, stir-fries, stews, and sauces, as well as bean purees and dips. (Some people use the liquid that canned beans are packed in, but I prefer to use water; for more about canned beans, see the sidebar on page 235.)

All of these benefits come with a minimal investment on your part: You rinse the beans and put them in a pot with water, bring the water to a low and steady bubble, and walk away. The result is an infinitely useful and versatile food that's full of fiber, protein, and other nutrients. If you have cooked beans handy, they quickly become the backbone of dips, spreads, stir-fries, and salads; they can also accent sandwiches, seafood, poultry, and meat dishes; and they are a constant companion to all sorts of cooked vegetable dishes.

---

1 pound dried beans, like chickpeas (see the variations for lentils and split peas)

Several bay leaves (optional)

2 teaspoons salt

1 teaspoon pepper

1 Rinse the beans under running water, picking through them for stones or debris. Soak them if you have time (see page 235), and put them in a large pot with enough cold water to cover by about 3 inches. Add the bay leaves if you're using them. Bring the water to a boil, then reduce the heat so bubbles are barely visible. Cover the pot tightly and let the beans cook undisturbed for 45 minutes.

2 Try a bean. If it's at all tender, add the salt and pepper. Make sure the beans are still covered by about 1 inch of water; add a little more if necessary. If the beans are still hard, don't add the seasonings yet and make sure they're covered by about 2 inches water; if not, add some.

3 Return the liquid to its very gentle bubble and cover. Now start checking for doneness every 10 to 15 minutes and, if necessary, add enough water to keep the beans just submerged. Small beans will take as little as 15 minutes more; older or larger beans can take up to an hour or more. If you haven't added salt and pepper yet, add them when the beans are just turning tender. Stop cooking when the beans are as firm or creamy as you like them. (I like beans more cooked than many people, but it's a matter of taste; for salads, firm and intact is often the way to go.) Taste and adjust the seasoning, and remove the bay leaves.

4 Now you have a few options: To use the beans as an ingredient in salads or other dishes where they need to be dry, or to finish all or some of them with one of the ingredients from the list on page 234, drain the beans and reserve the liquid separately (it's good to keep around if you end up making soup). To store the beans for later use, refrigerate them with their cooking liquid in an airtight container; you can always drain off the liquid later as needed. To freeze the beans, divide the beans and their liquid into individual or meal-size portions among airtight containers, leaving about an inch of space for expansion. To thaw the frozen beans, put them in the refrigerator overnight or heat the frozen block in a pot over low heat or in a bowl in the microwave. (Cooked beans will keep in the fridge for up to 1 week and in the freezer for months.)

VARIATIONS

BIG-BATCH COOKED LENTILS, SPLIT PEAS, OR SPLIT BEANS This includes many of the legumes found in Indian and Asian markets. Follow the directions in the main recipe, but start checking the beans or peas after about 15 minutes. Split peas and split beans will break down quickly and inevitably become soupy. (But if you want lentils intact for salads or stir-fries, watch them like a hawk and drain them the instant they get tender, before they break open.) Drain, reserving the cooking liquid if you like, and run under cold water to stop their cooking.

BIG-BATCH COOKED BEANS IN A SLOW COOKER The good news is that it's almost impossible to overcook beans this way, especially if you have a programmable machine that you can set to warm if you're not going to be home. (The exceptions are lentils and split beans or peas, which become soupy relatively quickly; if that's not what you want, just cook them on the stove.) Follow the directions in the main recipe, setting the slow cooker on either high or low depending on your desired timeframe. If using high, start checking the beans after 2 hours, and

(recipe continues)

after that every 30 minutes or so. If using low, start checking after 6 hours; then if you get impatient and they still aren't done, switch the setting to high to finish them off quickly.

BIG-BATCH COOKED FRESH SHELL BEANS Chickpeas, edamame, black-eyed peas, fava, and cranberry beans are the most common beans sold fresh. Since these are delicious and increasingly available in specialty stores or farmers' markets, here's how to cook them: Shell the beans if still in the pods and follow the directions in the main recipe, but cover the beans with only about 1 inch water. Start checking them after 20 minutes and every 5 minutes thereafter.

BIG-BATCH COOKED FROZEN SHELL BEANS Lima, edamame, and fava beans are the most common that are sold frozen. One could argue that they cook so quickly, why bother to do a big batch? Because like everything else, you'll eat them if they're ready to go. Follow the directions in the main recipe, but cover the beans with only about 1 inch of water. Start checking them after 5 minutes and every minute or so thereafter. (Or cook them in just ½ inch water in a covered dish in the microwave set on high, and start checking after 1 minute, and thereafter in 30-second intervals.)

WAYS TO FLAVOR COOKED BROWN RICE, WHOLE GRAINS, OR BEANS

Rather than season a whole pot of grains or beans the same way, I suggest adding ingredients a serving (or meal) at a time to keep things fresh and interesting. Try the following ingredients—alone or in combination. Note that flexible and "treat" ingredients should be used mindfully; see the pantry tables starting on page 35.

- Chopped fresh tomatoes
- Leftover cooked vegetables, like greens or peppers
- Chopped fresh herbs or crumbled dried herbs
- Any vinaigrette
- Soy sauce (more or less)
- Olive oil
- Sesame oil
- Spice blends, like curry or chili powder
- Minced chile, ginger, or garlic

- Hot sauce
- Balsamic or any wine vinegar
- Chopped toasted nuts or seeds
- Toasted unsweetened shredded coconut
- Butter (naturally!)
- Cooked crumbled bacon or sausage
- Mashed anchovies
- Grated Parmesan cheese
- Crumbled feta or blue cheese, or queso fresco

BEANS MADE SIMPLE

Like grains, beans are virtually interchangeable with one another in recipes, so I'm always on the lookout for legumes I haven't tried. In the years since I've been eating VB6 there's been an explosion in beans, from local sources as well as from around the world. So rather than overwhelming you with details about the dozens of different kinds, I hope this general information will encourage you to be on the lookout for those that are both familiar and new to you and that you explore their many tastes and textures.

DRIED BEANS

Your supermarket probably has more beans than ever before, but if it's the more exotic heirloom and specialty varieties you're after, try shopping the bulk sections in gourmet or natural food stores, or search online. (It's amazing how many local and regional sources you'll find.)

I rarely soak dried beans anymore; it takes only a little longer to cook unsoaked beans and the window of doneness is bigger so you can control the texture without watching the pot like a hawk. But if you are planning ahead, or are leaving the house (or going to sleep), submerging the beans in several inches of water for up to 12 hours will shorten their cooking time. Then to use soaked beans in the Big-Batch recipe (page 232), you should start by covering them in 2 (rather than 3) inches of water and start checking them after 30 minutes. Other than that, there's no change in the cooking directions, amount of attention (or real advantage).

FRESH (SHELL) BEANS

I can't say it enough: If you see 'em, grab 'em. Then see the variation after the main recipe on page 232 for directions on how to cook them.

CANNED BEANS

You've got to have at least a couple cans in the pantry at all times, even if you cook a pot of beans almost every week, as I do. It's better than being caught without. And if you look at a recipe and think *I'll never make my own beans*, then you'd better buy big cans and stock up. The variety of canned beans will never compare to what's available dried, but the selection—and quality—is good and always getting better, especially in natural food stores. Look for cans that say "BPA Free," which means the lining isn't coated in a type of plastic that might be toxic. And since canned beans are packed in a thick, often quite salty liquid, I always recommend you rinse and drain them well before using them in recipes.

FROZEN BEANS

I love the texture of frozen beans; they're the next best thing to fresh. Unfortunately, the types available are limited: Edamame, lima and fava beans, black-eyed peas, and sometimes chickpeas are about all you ever see, but they're all quite different. They also cook much faster than their dried counterparts and tend to stay intact longer. (See the variation after the main recipe on page 232 for cooking instructions.)

PICO DE GALLO

MAKES 4 servings   TIME 30 minutes

Fresh tomato salsa—or pico de gallo—has the power to transform plain pasta, grains, meat, chicken, fish, even eggs; it works as a side, a topping, a sauce, a dip, or all alone, eaten like gazpacho. And this is one of the most accommodating recipes I know: Change the tomatoes to another fruit or vegetable, vary the herb (or add spice), try a different kind of onion (or ginger). After checking out the main formula here, explore the variations and ideas that follow. No matter what you do, finish with a big squeeze of lime, which will unite everything perfectly.

6 tomatoes (about 2 pounds), chopped

1 small red onion, chopped

1 or 2 fresh hot chiles (like jalapeño), seeded if you like, minced

2 teaspoons minced garlic

1 cup chopped fresh cilantro (about 1 large bunch)

¾ teaspoon salt

¼ teaspoon black pepper

3 tablespoons fresh lime juice, or more to taste

1   Put the tomatoes in a large bowl with the onion, chile, garlic, cilantro, salt, and pepper. Stir once or twice.

2   Add the lime juice, then taste and adjust the seasoning, adding more juice if you like. Pico de gallo is best if you can let it sit at room temperature for 5 to 15 minutes so the flavors meld. (You can make it up to 2 hours ahead of time and refrigerate it; bring it back to room temperature before serving.)

VARIATIONS

GREEN PICO Use tomatillos instead of tomatoes and 4 scallions instead of the onion.

PINEAPPLE PICO Use 1 large (or two small) pineapple instead of the tomatoes, 1 tablespoon minced ginger instead of the garlic, and ½ cup chopped fresh mint instead of the cilantro.

PEACH PICO Substitute peaches for the tomatoes and fresh basil for the cilantro. Try lemon instead of lime juice.

ORANGE-CHILE PICO Perfect in winter when good tomatoes are scarce. Peel and chop about 2 pounds oranges, removing the seeds and tough bits of membrane. Use them instead of the tomatoes. Try a pinch of ground red chile or cayenne instead of the fresh chiles and herbs.

PICO DE GALLO WITH CORN Fantastic, but only when corn is in season and picked within a couple days of eating so it's fresh enough to eat raw. Replace 2 tomatoes with kernels cut from 2 ears of corn.

MORE IDEAS

Add avocado to the main recipe or any of the variations. • Instead of the tomatoes, try watermelon, plums, mangos, papayas, cherries, radishes, celery, or fennel. • Vary the aromatics: Shallots, scallions, onions, ginger, and garlic are all interchangeable.

NUT BUTTERS

MAKES 8 servings (or more)   TIME 5 minutes

If you have a food processor, you can make nut butter. You'll be amazed at how easy it is and how much more intense and fresher it tastes. (Once you grind nuts, their oils react with oxygen and can more quickly become rancid.) You can make nut butters from any nut, toasted or raw; all are good and, as you can imagine, all are different.

To toast the nuts before grinding, put them in a large dry skillet over medium heat. Cook, shaking the pan occasionally to turn them, until they smell fragrant and become as light or dark as you like (keeping in mind that the darker the color, the more intense and potentially bitter the flavor). This takes anywhere from 5 to 15 minutes depending on the nut (or seed) you use. Remove them from the pan immediately so they don't continue cooking, but wait to grind them until they cool a bit.

2 cups almonds, peanuts, cashews, or other nuts

1 teaspoon salt (optional)

Put the nuts in a food processor with the salt if you're using it and turn the machine on. Let it keep running until a paste forms. Stop to scrape down the sides of the bowl occasionally and add water, a few drops at a time, until you get the consistency you want. Transfer to a clean jar (will store in the fridge for up to a few weeks).

VARIATIONS

FRUIT AND NUT BUTTER Lowers the calorie density considerably and makes an excellent—but less thick—spread for morning toast. Try this with strawberries, raspberries, blackberries, blueberries, mangos, peaches, plums, figs, or cherries. Pulse 1 cup of whatever nut you like into a coarse meal, add 1 cup chopped fresh or thawed frozen fruit and 1 tablespoon fresh lemon juice, and let the machine run until the mixture is smooth. Refrigerate what you don't use right away (it will keep for up to 3 days).

COCONUT NUT-AND-FRUIT BUTTER Follow the variation above, only use ½ cup toasted or untoasted unsweetened shredded coconut to replace half the nuts.

SOY AND NUT BUTTER Savory and so good. Add 2 tablespoons soy sauce to the food processor before pureeing the nuts.

MORE IDEAS

Remember to consider unexpected nuts—and combinations: Try macadamia, pine nuts, walnuts, or pecans, for example. • Season the nut and seed butters with spices like cinnamon, cumin, nutmeg, or ginger; or blends like curry or chili powder or five-spice powder.

ALL-PURPOSE TOMATO SAUCE

MAKES eight 1¼-cup servings   TIME About 90 minutes

Marinara sauce—and that's what this is, essentially—is the basis for an array of sauces; see the variations below. You can make a half batch if you prefer, though this freezes so well I don't see why you'd bother. It takes just as much time (and only slightly more work) to ensure you have plenty on hand at all times. And there is no more useful cooked sauce.

2 tablespoons olive oil

1 onion, chopped

2 tablespoons minced garlic

1 teaspoon salt

½ teaspoon pepper

Red chile flakes, to taste

Two 28-ounce cans diced tomatoes, with their juice

1 cup chopped fresh basil, or ½ cup chopped fresh parsley (optional)

1 Put the oil in a large pot over medium heat. When it's hot, add the onion and garlic, ½ teaspoon of the salt, the pepper, and the red chile flakes if you're using it. Cook, stirring occasionally, until the vegetables soften, 3 to 5 minutes.

2 Add the tomatoes and the remaining ½ teaspoon salt, and adjust the heat so the mixture bubbles steadily. Cook, stirring occasionally, until the tomatoes break down, the vegetables become very soft, and the mixture thickens, 15 to 20 minutes. If the mixture looks too thick, stir in a splash of water.

3 Stir in the herb, if you're using it; taste and adjust the seasoning and serve. (Or store, tightly covered, in the refrigerator for up to several days, or in the freezer for up to several months.)

VARIATIONS

TOMATO SAUCE WITH LOTS OF VEGGIES Hearty, with a piece of vegetable in every bite. Increase the olive oil to ¼ cup and add another onion if you'd like. In Step 1, add 1 pound chopped mushrooms, 4 chopped carrots, and 2 chopped red or green bell peppers to the pot along with the onion and garlic. Cook, stirring occasionally, until the vegetables are soft and all of their liquid has evaporated, 25 to 30 minutes. Then continue with the recipe.

TOMATO SAUCE WITH GREENS You control the texture here. Remember that tender leaves like spinach or arugula are going to cook a lot faster than sturdy greens like escarole or collards. (Chard or cabbage falls somewhere in between.) Chop 1½ pounds any type of greens, stems and all. For silky tender greens that melt into the sauce—or perfectly tender sturdy greens—add them when you add the tomatoes in Step 2. For tender greens with a little more body, add them to the tomato sauce 2 or 3 minutes before it's done and cook, stirring occasionally, until they're as soft as you like.

COOKED RED SALSA (SALSA ROJA) Substitute red or white onions for the yellow onion, and add 2 chopped poblano chiles or 1 minced jalapeño chile (seeded if you'd like) along with the onion and garlic in Step 1. Use fresh cilantro instead of the basil. Let cool to room temperature or refrigerate until chilled. Squeeze in a little lime juice and the chopped cilantro before serving.

COOKED GREEN SALSA (SALSA VERDE) Follow the variation above, only use canned tomatillos instead of the tomatoes.

MAKHANI The tomato sauce of India, a winner when served over brown basmati rice. These directions work with either the main recipe or the loaded-with-vegetables variation. Substitute ½ cup coconut milk (reduced-fat is fine) for the olive oil. Just before adding the tomatoes in Step 2, stir 1 tablespoon curry powder into the onion mixture and cook, stirring constantly until fragrant, no more than a minute. Use fresh cilantro or mint for the basil.

MEATY TOMATO SAUCE Make either the main recipe or the loaded-with-vegetables variation. Start Step 1 by browning 1 pound ground beef, pork, chicken, turkey, lamb, or chopped or bulk sausage in the olive oil. Once it loses its pink color, drain off whatever fat you'd like (or not), add the vegetables, and continue with the recipe.

TOMATO SAUCE WITH CHICKEN Make either the main recipe or the loaded-with-vegetables variation. Start Step 1 by searing 1 pound boneless, skinless breasts or thighs (or 2 pounds bone-in chicken parts) in the oil. When browned all over—it doesn't need to be cooked all the way through—remove from the pan, add the vegetables, and cook according to the directions in the main recipe or the loaded-with-vegetables variation. When you add the tomatoes in Step 2, return the chicken to the pan at the same time so they cook together. The sauce is ready when the tomatoes break down and the meat is no longer pink, 15 to 30 minutes depending on the cut of chicken.

TOMATO SAUCE WITH SHRIMP OR SQUID Perfect as a pasta sauce or to serve over rice or toasted bread. Make either the main recipe or the loaded-with-vegetables variation. When the sauce is ready after Step 2, stir in 1 pound peeled shrimp or sliced squid. Cook, stirring occasionally until the seafood just turns opaque, 3 to 5 minutes.

MORE IDEAS

Try different fresh and dried herbs or spices, or add a splash of red or white wine.

TOFU TRIANGLES

MAKES 4 main-dish or 8 snack-size servings   **TIME** About 1 hour, almost entirely unattended

A vegan-ish diet is infinitely more interesting if it includes tofu, and tofu is infinitely more interesting if you add flavor—few things are as bland as tofu—or make it chewier. So much energy is spent to change blocks of tofu from a plain white mass into something more universally appealing. (See sidebar on page 113 for all you need to know about this remarkable and ancient food.)

Even though I happen to like tofu raw and include a few recipes for it that way, I especially enjoy it after the moisture is removed; if it develops a crust in the process, all the better. You can buy pressed tofu (if you can find it), but it's usually overly processed; you can easily press it yourself by sandwiching a block under a weighted pan (which slowly forces the water to leach out) or freezing it (which lets you squeeze the water out easily as it thaws).

Here are several simple treatments of tofu designed to help put more of it into your day. What they have in common is the contrast between a toothsome, slightly browned exterior and their custardy, almost egglike interior, as well as a pleasant, mildly beany taste that is good alone but also works with all sorts of seasonings. Chop or slice any of them into stir-fries, stews, soups, or salads; turn them into sandwiches; or eat them out of hand as snacks (they travel well and keep for days).

2 pounds firm tofu
(2 blocks)

½ teaspoon salt (optional)

1   Heat the oven to 300°F. Set the tofu block on one of its sides and cut it in half so that you have two rectangles, each about 1 inch thick. Cut each rectangle diagonally into 4 triangles about 1 inch thick.

2   Spread the tofu on a large baking sheet and transfer to the oven. Cook undisturbed until the triangles develop a browned crust and start to separate from the pan, 45 to 60 minutes, depending on how dry you want them. Sprinkle with the salt now if you'd like, or wait to season the tofu until you're ready to eat it. Let the triangles cool a bit before removing from the pan. (They might stick a bit in places but are easily pried free with a spatula.) To serve, cut the tofu into cubes or sticks of any size; or snack on the triangles whole.

VARIATIONS

TOFU TRIANGLES IN THE MICROWAVE Requires a little more attention but only a fraction of the time. Put the triangles on a microwave-safe plate lined with towels. Cook on high, stopping to turn and rotate the triangles a couple of times, until the tofu browns a little and looks fairly dry, 10 to 20 minutes depending on how firm and dry you want them.

EVEN CRISPER-AND MORE-TOFU TRIANGLES Perfect for snacking. Cut each triangle in half horizontally so you have 16 thin triangles, each about ½ inch thick. Cook in the oven or microwave according to the directions in the main recipe or variation above. They'll be ready in about half the time.

WHOLE ROASTED TOFU This is so great basted with vinaigrette, or even a little barbecue sauce or ketchup, during the last 10 minutes of roasting. Or try rubbing the blocks all over with a spice blend before popping them in the oven. Heat the oven to 350°F. Put the tofu blocks on the prepared sheet a few inches apart. Roast undisturbed until the blocks are browned, blistered in spots, and a bit shrunken, about 1 hour. Let cool completely before slicing as thin or thick as you like.

TOFU CROUTONS Crunchy on the outside, soft on the inside. Heat the oven to 350°F and line a rimmed baking sheet with foil or parchment. Cut the tofu blocks into 1-inch cubes and spread the pieces out on the baking sheet. Cook undisturbed until they shrink and brown, about 1 hour. They'll release easily from the pan as they cool.

MORE IDEAS

As it comes straight from the oven (or microwave), splash the tofu with soy sauce, you'll need only a little salt, if any. • Season the warm tofu with curry or chili powder, or five-spice powder (or any spice or seasoning blend).

VEGANNAISE

MAKES **8 servings**　　TIME **10 minutes**

I've been making my own mayonnaise for at least 30 years, and I still make it often, when I crave its richness. For an everyday dip or spread, though, I turn to this eggless version based on silken tofu. The base recipe is a simple and excellent enhancement for sandwiches and dressings, and when you start varying and adding ingredients, it's good enough to fool even a mayo aficionado like me.

8 ounces silken tofu (about 1 cup)

3 tablespoons olive oil

2 tablespoons cider vinegar

2 teaspoons Dijon mustard

¼ teaspoon salt

1 Put all the ingredients in a blender and puree, stopping once or twice to scrape down the sides of the container with a rubber spatula, until the tofu is completely smooth and evenly colored. This could take several minutes; add 1 or 2 tablespoons of water if necessary to help the machine do its work.

2 Taste and adjust the seasoning with more salt or vinegar if necessary. Serve right away (or transfer to a jar and refrigerate for up to 1 week).

VARIATIONS

GARLIC VEGANNAISE Also known as aïoli, the classic Mediterranean accompaniment to simply cooked vegetables, fish, chicken, or meat. Peel 2 to 8 garlic cloves, to taste, put them in the work bowl of the food processor, and pulse a few times to chop. Then add the remaining ingredients and proceed with the recipe.

LEMON OR LIME VEGANNAISE Tangy and bright like you won't believe. Use fresh lemon or lime juice instead of the vinegar and add 2 teaspoons grated lemon or lime zest.

MUSTARDY VEGANNAISE Bolster the Dijon with a tablespoon of coarse-ground mustard.

CREAMY BASIL SAUCE For dipping vegetables or as a dressing for salads and sandwiches. Use fresh lemon juice instead of the cider vinegar. Skip the Dijon. Add 1 packed cup fresh basil before pureeing.

ROASTED RED PEPPER VEGANNAISE Use white or red wine vinegar instead of the cider vinegar and skip the Dijon. Add 2 or 3 roasted red bell peppers to the work bowl and puree before adding the remaining ingredients (jarred peppers are fine here).

SOY VEGANNAISE Change a few ingredients for a versatile sauce that works with all sorts of Asian dishes. Use 2 tablespoons sesame oil instead of the olive oil, and rice vinegar instead of the cider vinegar. Keep the mustard if you'd like a little kick (or add 1 or more small fresh red chiles instead). Add 2 tablespoons soy sauce. Then puree.

MISO VEGANNAISE The mustard is delicious here, but for a milder sauce skip it. Use vegetable oil instead of the olive oil and fresh lemon juice instead of the vinegar. Add ¼ cup miso of any kind.

SAFFRON VEGANNAISE Just a pinch does it, but skip the mustard and use fresh lemon juice instead of the cider vinegar. Add it along with everything else.

MORE IDEAS

Instead of cider vinegar, you can use anything else acidic, like other vinegars (see page 23 for a rundown on the different options) or citrus juices. You can also leave it out altogether, but I think the mixture benefits from a little sharpness to mimic the tang of mayonnaise. • Add herbs. No more than 1 tablespoon fresh rosemary, oregano, thyme, or tarragon will do the trick. Or 2 tablespoons (or more) milder herbs like fresh mint, chives, chervil, or dill. • Add horseradish. Your call on how much, but start with 1 tablespoon and go from there. • Swap another condiment, like sriracha or another hot sauce, for the mustard. • Add spice (or a spice blend): Start with ¼ teaspoon, then add and taste as you puree. For blends like curry or chili powder, you'll need more like 1 tablespoon. • And remember to try the Chipotle "Mayo" (page 142), which is essentially the same idea as Vegannaise.

SEASONED SALT, YOUR WAY

MAKES **24 servings (½ cup)**   TIME **Less than 5 minutes**

You don't have to grind your own spices to make a good homemade spice blend; ground spices from a jar are just fine. But your own mix is fully customizable, depending on what proportions of ingredients you use: I put my spice mixes in small jam or recycled spice jars, but you can buy the kind with shaker inserts and lids if you'd like. Even a plate of plain steamed vegetables is instantly transformed into something special when you use your own seasoning.

¼ cup salt

2 tablespoon black pepper

1 tablespoon garlic powder

2 teaspoons sweet paprika

1 teaspoon ground allspice

Combine all the ingredients in a small jar or other container with a tight-fitting lid. Shake a few times. Store in a dark place and use within a few months.

VARIATIONS

YOUR OWN SMOKY SEASONED SALT One simple swap changes everything: Instead of the sweet paprika, use smoked paprika.

YOUR OWN MUSTARD SALT It's got a kick. Use 1 tablespoon dry mustard instead of the paprika and allspice.

YOUR OWN WASABI SALT The heat creeps, but in a good way. Use 1 tablespoon wasabi powder instead of the paprika and allspice.

YOUR OWN NORI SALT For a subtle brininess, instead of the garlic, paprika, and allspice, toast 4 sheets nori seaweed in a 400°F oven until dried and crisp, but not too brown, 3 to 5 minutes. Let cool, crumble, then combine with the salt and pepper and store as described in the main recipe.

YOUR OWN CHILI POWDER Or, more accurately, ground red chile, since the key here is to grind dried chiles. Ancho chiles are the easiest to find and they have a mild heat factor but moderately intense smokiness; dried chipotle chiles will be much hotter and smokier. (Note that there's no salt here so you can add it as you go.) Combine 4 tablespoons ground ancho chile with 1 teaspoon cayenne, 1 teaspoon black pepper, 4 teaspoons cumin, and 2 teaspoons ground coriander.

HERBES DE PROVENCE SALT Great when you don't have fresh herbs in the house. Omit the garlic, paprika, and allspice from the main recipe. Combine 1 teaspoon each dried rosemary, thyme, oregano, basil, marjoram, and fennel seed with the salt and pepper.

LEMON-PEPPER SALT Instead of the garlic, paprika, and allspice, use 2 tablespoons store-bought dried lemon zest.

ADOBO SEASONING Combine 2 tablespoons salt with 2 tablespoons garlic powder, 2 tablespoons black pepper, 2 teaspoons cumin, 1 tablespoon dried oregano, and 1 tablespoon turmeric (for color more than anything).

MUSHROOM SALT Put 1 ounce dried porcini, shiitake, morel mushrooms, or a combination, in a blender and pulse until coarse and the mushrooms are in flakes. Mix with ¼ cup salt. Use this to top sautéed vegetables, soups, pastas, or sandwiches.

FAST AND FLAVORFUL VEGETABLE STOCK

MAKES more than 2 quarts   TIME About 45 minutes

Like anything that comes in a box or a can, store-bought stock is undeniably convenient. And also like most prepared foods, it's not nearly as good as when you take the time to make it yourself. In fact, prepared vegetable stock is so bland that if I don't have time to make my own, I usually just use water (which is almost always an option in the recipes here).

The issue always boils down to time. But it's so easy to flavor water in a hurry with a mere handful of high-impact ingredients like mushrooms, tomato paste, and soy sauce, all of which have lots of *umami*, or "savoryness," that there's really no excuse not to. Since stock will keep in the fridge for a week or in the freezer for months, I encourage you to invest in a big pot and double (or triple) this recipe, then sock some away for the future. You can portion the stock into small containers for individual uses, or freeze it in ice cube trays to use in sauces and stir-fries.

1 large onion, quartered

4 carrots, cut into chunks

2 celery stalks, cut into chunks

1 pound button mushrooms, trimmed but left whole

4 (or more) whole garlic cloves, unpeeled, crushed

1 bunch fresh parsley, stems and leaves

4 fresh thyme sprigs, or a big pinch of dried

1 teaspoon whole black peppercorns

4 bay leaves

¼ cup tomato paste

¼ cup soy sauce

½ teaspoon salt, plus more to taste

Black pepper, to taste

1   Combine everything in a stockpot with 3 quarts of water. Bring to a boil and adjust the heat so the mixture bubbles steadily but gently. Cook until the vegetables are tender, about 30 minutes. (If you are in a hurry, you can stop cooking after 20 minutes; if you have a little extra time, let it simmer for 1 hour, go for it; the flavor will deepen and improve.)

2   Strain the stock, using a spoon to press on the vegetables to extract as much liquid as possible, then taste and add more salt and pepper if you like. Use right away or cool before storing.

VARIATIONS

SLOWER (BUT EVEN MORE FLAVORFUL) VEGETABLE STOCK Roast the onion, carrots, celery, mushrooms, and garlic in a 450°F oven, stirring occasionally, until brown, 30 to 45 minutes. Transfer the roasted vegetables to the stockpot and proceed with the recipe, simmering for 30 minutes or longer.

INTENSE MUSHROOM STOCK To the pot of vegetables in Step 1 add 1 cup dried porcini mushrooms. This is perfect when you want to create meatiness without using meat. But it's got a distinctive mushroom flavor, so if that's too pronounced for your purpose, stick with the main recipe or first variation.

STOCK WITH JUST A LITTLE SOMETHING That something being some sort of meat, fish, poultry, or the like. What you want to do is flavor the stock to enhance or amplify—rather than clash with—whatever you're using it for. So avoid combining meats; keep that in mind and you'll be fine. To the pot of vegetables in Step 1, add up to 4 ounces of the following: shrimp; fish fillets or steaks, clams or mussels; or boneless beef, chicken, pork (or ham or pork sausage), or lamb. Or toss in a handful of shrimp shells; some fish bones; a few chicken bones (especially those from the back and wings); or a big beef, pork, ham, or lamb bone.

MORE IDEAS

Add heat to the stock by including 1 or more small fresh chiles with the vegetables. Jalapeño, serrano, Fresno, or Thai bird are all good choices. • Add smokiness by including 1 or more dried chiles with the vegetables. Chipotle, ancho, and pasilla will all work—and come with varying degrees of heat. • Brighten the stock with a halved lemon, lime, or orange in the pot along with the vegetables. • Sweeten the stock—just a bit—with a cinnamon stick or a few cardamom pods, or try balsamic vinegar instead of the soy sauce. • If you don't have the parsley, use an extra teaspoon or so of dried herbs.

DASHI

MAKES about 2 quarts   TIME 15 minutes

During years of traveling, reporting, and cooking with others, I've learned to make dashi—the broth that is the backbone of Japanese cooking. Using dashi instead of water in miso broths results in a deeply complex but subtle flavor. And it's excellent for sipping like tea.

Dashi can be made several different ways. They're all ridiculously easy, all versatile, all delicious. It doesn't take many ingredients either, and you may be able to find them in your supermarket. If not, they're readily available in all Japanese and many other Asian markets and natural food stores. First is dried kombu, the seaweed we call kelp. It looks like a piece of dark green fruit leather with a salty crust. Next is bonito, a type of dried fish that's usually sold in the form of flakes called "shaved bonito." Either one or both are what give dashi its distinctive light and briny taste.

1 piece kombu (dried kelp)
4 to 6 inches long

½ cup bonito flakes

1 Put 9 cups water in a large pot with the kelp over medium heat. Don't let the mixture boil; just as bubbles start to rise from the bottom of the pan, turn off the heat and remove the kelp. (You can use the kelp in salads and stir-fries like any other vegetable.)

2 Immediately add the bonito flakes, stir, and let sit for 3 to 5 minutes, then strain. Use the dashi right away (or refrigerate for up to 2 days).

VARIATIONS

KOMBU DASHI Vegan and even more subtle, without any hint of fish. Omit the bonito flakes. The dashi is ready to use when you remove the seaweed in Step 1.

COLD WATER DASHI This works for the main recipe or the variations, but requires some advance thought. Put the kelp and/or bonito flakes in 2 quarts cold water and let sit on the counter for 6 to 8 hours. Strain and use or store as you would hot-water steeped dashi.

MORE IDEAS

To sweeten dashi, add mirin (sweet rice wine, readily available in supermarkets), maple syrup, or honey, 1 tablespoon at a time to taste. • To sharpen the flavor of dashi, add several slices of fresh ginger along with the kombu or bonito. (No need to peel it.) • To deepen the taste, add up to ¼ cup soy sauce to the dashi when you use it.

VB6 BREAD, SIX WAYS

MAKES **8 servings**   TIME **At least 1 hour**

We may not be able to live by bread alone, but no one should have to live without it. Since true whole-grain bread can be hard to find, the best alternative is often to just make it yourself. Fortunately, it's not that difficult (and not even that time-consuming) and it's incredibly good: hearty and deeply flavored, with a satisfying crumb that is equally appealing with salads and soups as it is topped with vegetables for quick handheld meals.

The main recipe here is for a cracker-like flatbread, which is fast and easy. The variations take the same dough and turn it into many entirely different things. See the sidebar on page 251 for how to make different kinds of breadcrumbs.

3 cups whole wheat flour, plus more for dusting

1 teaspoon instant yeast

1 teaspoon salt

1 cup warm water, plus more as needed

2 teaspoons olive oil

1   Combine the flour, yeast, and salt in a food processor. Turn the machine on and add the water and 1 teaspoon oil through the feed tube. Process until the dough becomes a barely sticky, easy-to-handle ball, about 30 seconds. If it's too dry, add more water a tablespoon at a time, and process for another 10 seconds. If it's too wet (unlikely), add more flour 1 tablespoon at a time. Turn the dough out onto a lightly floured surface, knead it a few times into a ball, and cover with a clean towel until it almost doubles in size, anywhere from 30 minutes to 2 hours depending on the temperature of your room.

2   Heat the oven to 500°F. Put a piece of parchment paper on your work surface and grease the paper with the remaining 1 teaspoon oil. Roll out the dough on the parchment until it's about ⅛ inch thick (the shape doesn't really matter). Carefully transfer the paper and dough to an ungreased baking sheet.

3   Bake, reversing the baking sheet once, until the bread is golden and crisp, and has puffed up slightly, 10 to 12 minutes. Cut the bread into 8 pieces, or tear it at the table. Serve hot, warm, or at room temperature. (Whatever you don't eat in a day or two, wrap in foil and store in the freezer. To reheat later, put the still-wrapped frozen bread in a 300°F oven until it thaws and warms, 20 to 30 minutes.)

(recipe continues)

VARIATIONS

SANDWICH BREAD Denser and smaller than commercial loaves, and ideal for thin slices that are perfect for all kinds of open-face and closed sandwiches. Grease a 9 by 5-inch loaf pan with 1 teaspoon olive oil. When the dough has risen after Step 1, flatten it into a rectangle, then fold the long sides into the middle so that you have a loose roll about the size of the pan and pinch the edges of dough together at the seam. Put the dough in the pan, seam side down, and tuck the short ends underneath so it fits in the pan. Press the dough firmly to spread to the corners of the pan as best you can. Cover with a towel and let rest until it puffs up again, 30 to 60 minutes. Heat the oven to 350°F. Bake until the top is crusty and the inside is cooked through (the internal temperature should be about 210°F), 40 to 50 minutes. Let cool for 10 minutes before inverting onto a wire rack, then cool thoroughly before slicing.

BREADSTICKS Heat the oven to 400°F. Once the dough has risen and been rolled as described in Steps 1 and 2, slice the rectangle into equal pieces about as wide as you want your breadsticks to be. Pressing gently on the dough with both hands on a flat work surface, roll out each piece so that it's the same thickness throughout, as long or short as you want; dust the surface lightly with more whole wheat flour to keep the breadsticks from sticking. When they're the size you want, put them back on the parchment paper and transfer to the oven. Bake, turning (or rolling) a few times, until they're golden on the outside and cooked through in the middle, 8 to 10 minutes for ¼ inch thick, 10 to 12 minutes for ½ inch, and 12 to 14 minutes for 1 inch. Serve hot, warm, or at room temperature.

RUSTIC CRUSTY BREAD Heat the oven to 450°F. Put a 2- to 3-quart cast-iron, enamel, all stainless steel, or ceramic pot in the oven while it heats. When the oven is hot, carefully remove the pot from the oven and gently put the round of dough into the pot. Cover the pot and return to the oven. Bake for 20 minutes, then remove the lid and bake until the loaf is beautifully browned, another 15 to 20 minutes. If at any point the bread smells like it's burning, lower the heat. Remove the bread from the pot and let cool completely on a wire rack before slicing.

FOCACCIA After the dough has risen in Step 1, smear a large baking sheet with 1 tablespoon olive oil. Press the dough into the pan, leaving it ¼ to ½ inch thick; dimple the top with your fingertips and sprinkle with salt, pepper, a tablespoon chopped fresh rosemary, and another tablespoon olive oil. Cover with a towel and let the dough sit until it puffs nicely, 30 to 60 minutes, depending on the heat of the room. After the dough has been resting about 15 minutes, heat the oven to 500°F. Bake until golden all over and springy to the touch, 15 to 20 minutes. Let cool in the pan before cutting into squares or breaking into pieces.

CROUTONS Make as large or as small a batch as you'd like, with freshly made bread or whatever leftover bits and pieces you have handy. Heat the oven to 400°F. Cut the bread into cubes with sides at least ½ inch thick. Spread the bread out on a rimmed baking sheet without overlapping. Bake, shaking the pan to turn the cubes until lightly browned and crisp all over, 10 to 15 minutes. Let cool and serve right away (or store in an airtight container for up to several days).

MORE IDEAS

Flavor the dough: After it comes together in the food processor, fold in chopped fresh or crumbled dried herbs; ground spices; minced garlic, ginger, chiles, olives, or dried tomatoes; or even chopped nuts. • Add more olive oil, either to the dough during mixing or by brushing a bit more onto the top of the loaves, breadsticks, or croutons just before baking. • Season the tops of the flatbread, breadsticks, or focaccia: Treat it like pizza and scatter any of the ingredients above on top once the dough is in the pan. Or try an assortment of chopped raw or cooked vegetables, olives, capers, roasted red peppers, or caramelized onions. The ingredients will stick better with a coating of olive oil first, but it's not essential. Just make sure to use a light hand with the topping; if you weight down the dough too much, it won't puff up as it should.

BREADCRUMBS

With VB6 you probably won't be eating as much bread as you have in the past. So get in the habit of freezing what's left of a loaf before it gets stale. Then whenever you get some critical mass socked away, make a batch of breadcrumbs, one of two ways:

Fresh Breadcrumbs: Figure a 1-pound whole-grain loaf will make 3 to 4 cups crumbs. This technique is perfect when you have a chunk of leftover bread you don't know what to do with. If you have little bits, freeze them until you get enough to make at least a half batch. Tear or cut the bread into 2-inch pieces and put about half in a food processor. Pulse a few times to bust it, but then let the machine run just long enough to chop the bread as coarsely or finely as you'd like. (Stop the machine to peek frequently because it doesn't take long.) Transfer the crumbs to an airtight container and repeat with the remaining bread. Use right away or store at room temperature for up to 1 month (or freeze for up to 3 months). (Try frying these in a little olive oil until crisp and use them as a garnish for vegetables.)

Dried Breadcrumbs: Heat the oven to 350°F. Follow the steps above for fresh breadcrumbs, only after grinding the bread, spread the crumbs out evenly on a rimmed baking sheet; toast them, shaking the pan occasionally, until they're as light or dark as you'd like, 10 to 20 minutes, depending on how fine they are. Let them cool a bit before transferring them to an airtight container.

ACKNOWLEDGMENTS

In the year since the publication of the original VB6, part-time veganism, flexitarianism, the increasingly but not exclusively plant-based diet—whatever you want to call it—has become a common discussion. That VB6 and diets like it "work" is not in dispute. Whether I helped make this happen in some small part is not that important; what matters is that it's happening, and it's a really good thing.

Happily, not much has changed in my personal life in that year, so I can write a simpler and less dramatic series of thank-yous.

Kerri Conan, my book-writing partner of nearly ten years, has surpassed herself here, working under almost impossible deadline pressure while helping us maintain our usual high quality level. (I trust you will agree.) She had help from Daniel Meyer, now a longstanding part of my wonderful team, which during the past couple of years has included Suzanne Lenzer, Meghan Gourley, Elena Goldblatt, Jennifer Griffin (yay!), Eve Turow, Emily Saltz, and Reina Podell. The stunning photos in this cookbook are thanks to Quentin Bacon, with whom I first worked in 1996, if you can believe that, and who has gotten, if possible, even more talented (and more mellow) with age.

During the course of this year, the relationship between me and Clarkson Potter editor and publisher Pam Krauss—who has nothing to prove—has only grown stronger; we are doing the work we want to do, and you're holding it in your hands. Kate Tyler, whose life became a tad more complicated in 2013, admirably managed publicity for the first book, and (though she also has nothing to prove) will no doubt do it again; she was ably assisted by Anna Mintz, who has learned how to mood-manage me. There are a dozen other people at Potter who've worked hard with me in the last couple of years, including Carly Gorga, Donna Passannante, Maha Khalil, Mark McCauslin, La Tricia Watford, Kim Tyner, and Jessica Freeman-Slade.

As usual, Kerri and I owe big debts to the slimmed-down version of Sean Santoro and to Wendy and Kim Marcus.

I hope that I thank other friends and loved ones often enough so that it would be superfluous here.

For those of you who are new to VB6, welcome; you are making a good choice in starting. For those who are buying this cookbook for reinforcement after starting VB6 some time in the last year, thank you—you're going to love what's in here.

INDEX